Rethinking Our War on Drugs

Candid Talk about Controversial Issues

Gary L. Fisher

Foreword by William L. White

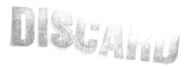

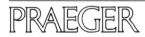

Westport, Connecticut
London

Library of Congress Cataloging-in-Publication Data

Fisher, Gary L.

    Rethinking our war on drugs : candid talk about controversial issues / Gary L. Fisher ;
    foreword by William L. White.

      p. ; cm.

    Includes bibliographical references and index.

    ISBN–13: 978–0–275–99026–8 (alk. paper)

    ISBN–10: 0–275–99026–5 (alk. paper)

    1. Drug control—United States.   2. Drug control—United States—History.
3. Drug abuse—United States—Prevention.   I. Title.

    [DNLM: 1. Drug and Narcotic Control—United States.   2. Public Policy—United
States.   3. Substance-Related Disorders—United States.]

  HV5825.F5653   2006

  363.450973–dc22   2006024491

British Library Cataloguing in Publication Data is available.

Copyright © 2006 by Gary L. Fisher

All rights reserved. No portion of this book may be
reproduced, by any process or technique, without the
express written consent of the publisher.

Library of Congress Catalog Card Number: 2006024491
ISBN: 0–275–99026–5

First published in 2006

Praeger Publishers, 88 Post Road West, Westport, CT 06881
An imprint of Greenwood Publishing Group, Inc.
www.praeger.com

Printed in the United States of America

∞™

The paper used in this book complies with the
Permanent Paper Standard issued by the National
Information Standards Organization (Z39.48–1984).

10 9 8 7 6 5 4 3 2 1

To Carole, you inspire me to be humble.

Contents

Foreword

Rethinking Our War on Drugs arrives at an interesting time in American political and cultural history. After a brief period of reform in the 1960s and 1970s (penalty reductions and diversion to treatment), alcohol and other drug problems have been restigmatized, demedicalized, and recriminalized under a philosophy of "zero tolerance" that has spanned Democrat and Republican administrations. A century ago, it appeared that the United States was moving toward a very consistent policy of prohibiting alcohol, tobacco, and the nonmedical use of opiates and cocaine. After brief state and national experiments with alcohol prohibition and local and state tobacco prohibition in the early twentieth century, new policies were forged, based on the notion of good drugs and bad drugs. Newly defined good drugs such as alcohol and tobacco were celebrated, commercialized, and aggressively promoted while bad drugs such as heroin and cocaine and later marihuana and hallucinogens were increasingly demonized and criminalized, with prescription psychoactive drugs existing on the border between these two worlds. Most of the policy debates of the past century have occurred within this enduring good drug–bad drug dichotomy. *Rethinking Our War on Drugs* is, among other things, a call to transcend this dichotomy.

There is a critical need to elevate the discussion of American drug policy, but several factors work against this. Individuals and families personally impacted by addiction are collectively silenced within the shame and stigma in which these problems have been culturally encased. At the same time, the existing framework of drug supply reduction and drug demand reduction feeds billions of dollars ($145 billion in the past 10 years) into institutional economies: innumerable governmental bodies, law enforcement agencies, the court systems, an evergrowing prison system, addiction treatment institutions, prevention agencies, and all the subindustries (e.g., equipment, training, research) that support them. One of the problems this creates is that nearly everyone professionally close to alcohol and other drug problems is financially rewarded within the current infrastructures that define cultural ownership of these problems. Sadly, those with alcohol and drug problems constitute a crop to be regularly harvested for institutional and personal profit. Such rewards buy considerable silence and limit open debate about drug policy. There are, however, voices that have broken and continue to break this silence.

American drug control policies have undergone critical analysis since the basic architecture of these policies was first established. The analysis of these policies has ranged from scholarly histories (e.g., Dr. David Musto's *The American Disease: Origins of Narcotic Controls*, 1973) through expert panels of the American Medical and Bar Associations to rhetorical diatribes (e.g., Thomas Szasz's *Ceremonial Chemistry*, 1974). Falling between these poles is a tradition of careful analysis suggesting that the intentions of these polices have not been met and have instead created unanticipated and quite harmful effects on individuals, families, communities, and the country as a whole. The most significant contributions within this latter tradition include Henry Williams' *Drug Addicts Are Human Beings* (1938), William Eldridge's *Narcotics and the Law* (1968), Rufus King's *The Drug Hang-up: America's Fifty Year Folly* (1972), Troy Duster's *The Legislation of Morality* (1972), Alfred Lindesmith's *The Addict and the Law* (1973), and such recent contributions as Dan Baum's *Smoke and Mirrors* (1996) and Michael Massing's *The Fix* (1998). Gary Fisher's *Rethinking Our War on Drugs*, in its critical analysis of the National Drug Control Strategy between 1996 and 2005, is the latest offering within this tradition of dissent.

Criticism of American drug policy has often come at a high price. Local and national politicians, judges, police chiefs, law enforcement officers, treatment specialists, and even surgeon generals as well as prestigious groups like the American Medical Association and the American Bar Association have paid high prices for their candor. The risks of financial punishment (e.g., withdrawal of government funding), political harassment, and professional scapegoating have been so great that only those in the most insulated positions (e.g., tenured professors at private universities) have risked the backlash of their published criticism of current drug policies. Future sacrifices are likely as momentum builds for a fundamental reevaluation of these policies. Those who claim the king is wearing no clothes (that the American drug policies have not and are not working) will be branded as misguided and dangerous and blackballed until the political winds shift. In the aftermath of that shift, today's provocateurs will be lauded as courageous visionaries. What will propel this shift more than any single factor is the emergence of a global village. As American citizens become more closely connected to the world community, their awareness of alternatives to our current drug policies will force a more critical examination and reevaluation of American policy. *Rethinking Our War on Drugs* is another straw on the back of American drug policy—another call for us to step back and rethink how we got into this war and how we can get out of it.

There are several things that commend this book. First, Fisher has a distinguished history of working within the existing policy framework. He brings no axe to grind about particular policy leaders or institutions. What follows are not the disgruntled words of a whistleblower, but the words of a reformer convinced that a better way must be found. Fisher argues not for a particular policy or single strategy but for fearless scrutiny and dialog about present policies and their potential alternatives, including the most controversial and politically tabooed (from harm reduction, decriminalization, and legalization to increases in alcohol taxation). As a person in recovery, Fisher also brings the perspective of one who has experienced alcohol and other drug problems and their solutions at a most personal level. As an individual who has long chosen to use none of the drugs discussed in this book, his arguments cannot be discounted as the self-justifications of an active drug user (a suspicion often cast on those advocating changes in current drug policies). Fisher views our current predicament as a function of flawed policies rather than of inadequate resources, organizational malaise, or professional ineptitude. He is offering one of the most eloquent arguments to date (using the government's own established objectives and performance benchmarks) of what is becoming obvious to a growing number of citizens: American drug policies and strategies are impotent to achieve the noble goals to which they aspire.

There is a deep thread of irrationality within the history of American drug control policies. Presidents and Congress have repeatedly created expert panels only to chastise and ignore the reports of those panels when their recommendations are not politically palatable. It is time the American citizenry wrenched this issue from the politicians who exploit this issue and the equally rabid drug warriors and drug legalizers. It is time citizens in local communities across the country reclaimed their investment in this problem. There is some evidence that the citizenry is reaching this point of readiness. It is becoming increasingly clear that our renewed efforts to incarcerate our way out of alcohol and drug problems are failing. Citizens are disillusioned that illicit drugs are more available, more potent, and cheaper in local American communities in spite of billions of tax dollars that have gone into drug enforcement. Citizens are also looking more critically at the degree of effectiveness of both prevention programs and addiction treatment programs. Perhaps the time is right to revisit a policy discussion that began more than a century ago and led us down a path whose destination was unclear. It is not too late to re-chart that path, but it will take courage.

Alcohol and other drug problems have an importance that far surpass their harm to individuals and society. Policies related to these problems touch on some of the most critical issues in our society: race, social class, gender, the health of families and communities, intergenerational conflict, corporate greed, and America's relationships with other countries. The stakes involved in all of these are too important to tolerate continued policy inertia and cultural silence about the premises that lie beneath our current policies. This book is a report card on what we are doing in this policy arena and a bold call to reevaluate those policies. It is a reasoned call for conversation—a call to rethink not our goals of preventing and resolving these problems, but the strategies we are currently using to achieve those goals. Gary Fisher is challenging us to begin that conversation today and to not let anyone arbitrarily limit the options that we can include in that conversation. Let the conversation begin.

William L. White

Preface

The first time I realized that there was something terribly wrong with the National Drug Control Strategy was in 1993. While writing a textbook for substance abuse counseling classes, I came across some reports on the results of United States' efforts to stop the supply of illegal drugs that enter the country. From these reports, it did not appear that there had been any reduction in the supply of cocaine and heroin available in the United States. Frankly, this was shocking because, with all of the news reports about huge drug busts, I was sure that we were winning the "war" on illegal drug supplies. The United States was spending a lot of money on this and I believed that, with our technological advantages, we should be able to outsmart the criminal drug smugglers.

By 1997, I had been involved in federal programs designed to reduce the demand for illegal drugs for about 4 years. I had just been awarded a $1 million a year grant to develop one of five regional centers involving substance abuse prevention. While in Washington, D.C., for a meeting with federal officials and the other grant directors, we were given a preview of the new antidrug commercials that were going to be aired in the next 6 months. After watching these commercials, it was apparent that the prevention part of the National Drug Control Strategy was in trouble. I had worked in public schools as a psychologist for a number of years and was confident in my understanding of adolescent development. These commercials were doomed to fail. None of them had anything to do with alcohol use (the substance used the most by adolescents) and the content was inappropriate to impact young people. The other grant directors felt the same way.

In 2000, my home state of Nevada passed a medical marijuana law and in 2004, the state defeated a ballot initiative to legalize the possession of a small amount of this drug. During the campaigns for both of these laws, our state had frequent visits from federal officials from the Office of National Drug Control Policy, including the Drug Czars. During their speeches and press conferences, these officials exaggerated the dangers of marijuana, misrepresented research on the drug, and distorted information to fit their point of view.

After being a part of the National Drug Control Strategy for over 10 years, by 2004, I was convinced that our approach to drug policy was totally flawed. Through two administrations, one Democrat and one Republican, and countless meetings with federal officials, all I heard were recycled ideas, promises of progress when the data showed there was no progress, misinformation, and the waste of billions of dollars.

But, two events finally motivated me to write this book. The first was an initiative called the Strategic Prevention Framework State Incentive Grants funded by the Center for Substance Abuse Prevention in the Substance Abuse and Mental Health Administration, a part of Health and Human Services. These grants started in fiscal year 2004. They are awarded to states and are for $2.35 million a year for 5 years. Nineteen states were funded in fiscal year 2004, 5 in fiscal year 2005, and 12 to 15 more are planned for fiscal year 2006. These grants are designed to help states and communities develop and implement comprehensive, evidence-based prevention programs and strategies.

That may sound reasonable to you. However, in 1997, this same agency had a grant program called the State Incentive Grant. These grants provided $3 million a year for 3 years to states to help communities implement evidence-based prevention programs. Nearly every state eventually received one of these awards. So, after spending hundreds of millions of dollars on the State Incentive Grant program, the Center for Substance Abuse Prevention decided they hadn't done this the right way. So they are starting all over again, doing nearly the same thing, and spending hundreds of million dollars more. What do we have to show for this? Nothing. And, the federal officials who developed this new program have absolutely no idea about whether the new program will be anymore effective than the first one.

The second event that motivated me to write this book occurred about a year after this "new" initiative was announced. I was attending a meeting in Washington, D.C., for one of the grants in the center I ran. A high-level official in the Center for Substance Abuse Prevention told the representatives of the grants that we had to submit any materials we developed for clearance if the materials mentioned increasing alcohol excise taxes. As you will read in this book, increasing alcohol excise taxes is an effective method to reduce underage drinking. However, as this federal official told us, we have to be careful about advocating for increasing alcohol excise taxes because of pressure from the alcohol industry.

So, at the same time the Center for Substance Abuse Prevention is wasting hundreds of millions of taxpayer dollars on redundant programs that have not worked, this agency is saying that we can't recommend strategies that have been shown to be effective because the alcohol industry objects.

I decided that I needed to thoroughly document the failure of our National Drug Control Strategy and to suggest alternatives that, in my opinion, would make it more effective. The intent to this book is not to heap ridicule and criticism on the Office of National Drug Policy but to generate a dialog about how to manage the tremendous problem of alcohol and other drug abuse. If this book can help to stimulate this discussion, it will have been well worth the effort to write it.

Speaking of effort, I want to thank some of my colleagues for reviewing selected chapters of the book. Their suggestions were very helpful and I appreciate their support. However, they would prefer to remain anonymous because of their concern regarding the potential consequences of being associated with the criticism of federal funding sources. I also appreciate the objective review and suggestions from James A. Swartz, Associate Professor at the Jane Addams College of Social Work at the University of Illinois, Chicago. My brother, Michael Fisher, read every word of this manuscript and gave me uncensored feedback. I can always count on my older brother to be brutal. My wife and best friend, Carole Fisher, also read every word, several times. Although this was a tedious task, she did read carefully and forced me to be clearer than I tend to be. Carole also put up with my anxiety about the project. I am grateful for her ability to manage me.

Finally, I want to thank all the staff members at the Center for the Application of Substance Abuse Technologies at the University of Nevada, Reno. I was blessed with a group of talented and dedicated people. Most of them knew that I was working on a book and that the content was secret. Nothing in this book should detract from their hard work and professionalism. Part of the tragedy of our National Drug Control Strategy is that these people are constrained by the parochial perspective of policy makers. I hope this book contributes to providing them the freedom to accomplish what they are capable of.

The Battle Plan on the war on Drugs has failed

One

The War on Drugs: Is the Battle Plan Working?

Introduction

In 1988, Congress passed a law that created the Office of National Drug Control ∧ $?
Policy in order to develop and implement a national drug control strategy. At that
time, the price per gram of powder cocaine was $199.98. In 1996, the middle
of the Clinton administration, that same gram of cocaine cost $179.83. In the
second quarter of 2003 (the most current available data but nearly the middle of
the Bush administration), that gram of cocaine was $94.12 (all of the figures are
in 2002 constant dollars).[1] In the 15 years between 1988 and the middle of 2003,
Republican and Democratic administrations in the United States have spent over
$100 billion to reduce the supply of illegal[2] drugs such as cocaine in our country
because, according to the White House Office of National Drug Control Policy,
"... when supplies are disrupted, prices go up."[3] However, something must be
wrong because in spite of spending all of this money, the price of cocaine has
actually *fallen* more than 50 percent.   ↓50%

In 1991, 11.2 percent of young people in the 8th–12th grades had used an   1991–11.2%
illicit drug in the past month.[4] In 2005, 16.3 percent of the same age groups had   2005–16.3
used illicit drugs in this time period.[5] Over this 14-year period, the United States
has spent about $27 billion to prevent young people from using illicit drugs.
Something must be wrong because the rate of illicit drug use has *risen* nearly
50 percent.   ∧50%

As you will see in this book, the supply of cocaine that enters the United States
has not been significantly disrupted. Almost without exception, the supplies of
other illegal drugs have also remained at or above the levels at the beginning of the
War on Drugs. Furthermore, there is virtually no evidence that federal prevention

initiatives have had any impact on the illicit drug use patterns of young people or on the harm caused by illicit drug abuse. Therefore, it is not difficult to answer the question raised in the title of this chapter, "The War on Drugs: Is the Battle Plan Working?" With regard to the disruption of the supply of illegal drugs in the United States and the prevention of illicit drug use and abuse, the battle plan of the War on Drugs has failed.

In this book, all of the components of the War on Drugs will be examined. The strategies, initiatives, and activities that have been implemented will be critiqued by looking at the outcomes of these efforts. The results of all of our work to stop the flow of illicit drugs into the United States will be reviewed. Research results will be utilized to determine if our efforts in prevention and treatment have been wise. Controversial alternatives to our current policies (e.g., decriminalization, legalization, harm reduction, medicinal use of marijuana) that have always been rejected by federal officials will be critically explored.

The focus of this book will be on the National Drug Control Strategy (NDCS) of the United States in the last 10 years (1996–2005). There are several reasons to focus on this period. First, it spans Democratic (Clinton) and Republican (Bush) administrations. Both parties have followed similar paths. So this analysis is not biased toward or against any political philosophy. Second, this 10-year period includes the tenure of two significant Directors of the Office of National Drug Control Policy (i.e., Drug Czars). General Barry McCaffrey was Clinton's Drug Czar from 1996 to 2000 and John Walters began his tenure in the Bush administration in 2001 and is the current Drug Czar (as of June 2006). Furthermore, until 1994, ONDCP did not have the authority to establish budgets and allocate resources. Therefore, prior to this time, the Drug Czar had status but not much power. Finally, I am focusing on these 10 years because I have been personally involved in implementing aspects of our NDCS during this time period.

While this book is meant to be an objective analysis of our NDCS, I think it is important for readers to understand why I am writing this and if I have an "agenda." I am a professor at a public university in the West and was the director of a grant-funded center at this institution until July 1, 2006, when I asked to be reassigned to more traditional academic responsibilities.[6] In 1987, I volunteered to develop and teach a graduate class for counselors on drugs and alcohol. At the time, I was training school psychologists and I thought it would be fun to do something different. From my research in preparing to teach this course, I found out that there was grant money available in the substance abuse field and, in 1989, I received a grant from the U.S. Department of Education to provide training about alcohol and other drugs to undergraduates who were preparing to become teachers, and, 2 years later, another grant to help prevent substance abuse among learning disabled students in middle schools. In late 1993, I was able to secure a 5-year, $3 million grant from the Substance Abuse and Mental Health Services Administration (SAMHSA) in the U.S. Department of Health and Human Services. (SAMHSA is the primary federal agency that implements the NDCS in the areas of prevention and treatment.) That led to more grants and the development of a center at my university devoted to helping substance abuse prevention and treatment providers use evidence-based practices in their work. Since that first SAMHSA grant, my staff and I received somewhere in the neighborhood of $33 million in grants and contracts, mostly from SAMHSA. The center has over 50 employees located throughout the western United States, providing services to the 11 western states and the 6 Pacific jurisdictions.

As the recipient of federal grants, I have frequently attended meetings in Washington, D.C., where federal officials discuss our NDCS, particularly in regard to prevention and treatment. I have had the opportunity to talk to state officials, other grant recipients, and federal employees about our NDCS. Through the years, I have become acquainted with people who are connected to high-level federal officials involved with developing and implementing the NDCS.

In other words, I am an insider in the War on Drugs. I have been involved in the implementation of parts of the NDCS for over 12 years. I am not a disgruntled employee nor am I seeking revenge on any federal official or agency. On the contrary, the center I ran has been very successful in obtaining grant funding. I simply think it is time for those of us who are involved in the implementation of the NDCS to tell the public what is really happening.

For example, several years ago, the Director of the Center for Substance Abuse Treatment (an agency in SAMHSA), reprimanded me because we had sponsored Jocelyn Elders, former surgeon general, to speak at a conference. Dr. Elders had been fired by President Clinton because of her controversial comments, including saying that there should be a *discussion* about decriminalizing illegal drugs. The Director of the Center for Substance Abuse Treatment did not want any federal dollars to be spent on a speaker who could be associated with even suggesting that the U.S. government reexamine criminal penalties for illegal drug use. Other federal officials from this same agency have told my staff and me that we cannot have any training activity or develop any materials that use the term "harm reduction." Harm reduction is the concept of developing policies to reduce the harm caused by illicit drug use, such as allowing intravenous drug users to exchange dirty needles for clean ones. About a month before I started this book, I attended a meeting with federal officials in Washington, D.C. Bob Denniston, the individual who directs the $100 million National Youth Anti-Drug Media Campaign for ONDCP, told us that he must allow representatives from the alcohol industry to preview commercials that have any content on underage drinking before running these spots.[7] At this same meeting, we were told that we had to get approval for any training materials that mention increasing alcohol excise taxes as a method of reducing the harm caused by alcohol. We were told quite directly that this was due to pressure from the alcohol industry on Congress.

While these incidents and prohibitions may not strike you as catastrophic, they are indicative of a major barrier to making progress in our NDCS. If there are limits on what can be discussed and lobbying groups can censure information, these restrictions impact the ability of experts to creatively develop methods to improve our NDCS. As you will see in this book, alcohol and other drug abuse is a major societal problem. Our NDCS has basically used the same model over many years to deal with this problem. With some exceptions, this hasn't worked. It is impossible to know if alternative models will be more successful. However, it certainly makes sense to allow people with immense practical and professional knowledge to develop alternatives without restrictions due to biases, stereotypes, misinformation, and political agendas. A major purpose of this book is to advocate for this open exchange of ideas.

There is one other personal aspect I must mention. I am a recovering alcoholic and drug addict. After I had received my first large federal grant, I realized that my alcohol and drug use was out of control. I did not enter formal treatment but have utilized commonly known recovery programs for support. I am sharing this because there are groups who advocate for changing drug policies because their members want to be able to use currently illegal drugs without criminal penalties. I am not a member of or aligned with any of these groups. It would not change my behavior if marijuana or any other drug became legal. I have to abstain from alcohol and other drugs because I am an alcoholic/addict. However, I strongly believe that reasonable people have to be able to discuss decriminalization and legalization and there is a chapter on this topic.

Historical Origins of the War on Drugs[8]

The actual term "War on Drugs" can be traced back to 1971 during the Nixon administration. Due to a concern that many servicemen returning from Vietnam were addicted to heroin, Nixon appointed the first Drug Czar and created the Special Action Office for Drug Abuse Prevention and, in 1973, the Drug Enforcement Agency (DEA) was established. After Nixon resigned, Ford did not spend much time on drug issues. However, in 1975 a white paper was released by the Domestic Council Drug Abuse Task Force that recommended that supply and demand efforts be directed toward the most dangerous drugs. The paper called marijuana a low-priority drug. During his campaign, President Carter actually proposed the elimination of federal penalties for possession of one ounce or less of marijuana. However, due to the political realities of such a move and the other problems during his presidency, no real effort was made to follow through on this. When Reagan came to office, a cocaine and crack epidemic had begun in America. A great deal of media attention was directed toward the large cocaine seizures in Florida, with the drugs originating in Colombia and transported through Panama. Nancy Reagan began the "Just Say No" campaign in 1984. As the title of the campaign implies, this was a public relations effort to encourage young people to refuse to use illicit drugs. In this same year, an extremely large marijuana cultivation and processing center was destroyed in Mexico and a great deal of drug-related violence was occurring in Central America. After the death of Len Bias, a college basketball player who had just been drafted by the Boston Celtics and died after ingesting cocaine, public pressure to "do something" was at an all-time high. In response, Reagan signed the Anti-Drug Abuse Act of 1986. That bill included mandatory minimum sentences for drug offenses and differentiated penalties for selling powder cocaine from selling crack cocaine (e.g., 5 kilograms of powder cocaine = 10 years while 5 grams of crack cocaine = 5 years). In other words, a person selling 1/1,000 the amount of crack cocaine as powder cocaine received a prison sentence half as long as the cocaine dealer. So, small dealers of crack were likely to be sent to prison for years. The result of this was disparities in the racial composition of prison populations because African-Americans were much more likely than other races to be arrested for distributing small amounts of crack cocaine. In 1988, Reagan signed the Anti-Drug Abuse Act of 1988 which created the Office of National Drug Control Policy (ONDCP) to set priorities, implement a national strategy, and certify federal drug control budgets. The bill directed ONDCP to prevent young people from using illicit drugs, reduce the number of people using illicit drugs, and decrease the availability of illicit drugs.

In 1988, President George Herbert Walker Bush appointed William Bennett to head ONDCP. Bennett advocated making drug abuse socially unacceptable. Whereas the budget for ONDCP increased while Bennett was Drug Czar, two-thirds of the dollars were directed toward supply reduction and one-third to prevention and treatment. During the Clinton administration, Executive Order No. 12880 was implemented in 1993 and the Violent Crime Control and Law Enforcement Act of 1994 was passed. Through these measures, ONDCP was given responsibility for leading drug control policy and control of budgets and resources. The first Drug Czar in the Clinton administration was Lee Brown who served from 1993 to 1995. General Barry McCaffrey was confirmed as Drug Czar by the Senate in 1996, two days after Clinton nominated him. McCaffrey's experience in the alcohol and other drug field was as commander of the U.S. military's Southern Command where he battled drug smugglers.[9] General McCaffrey did not like the analogy of "war" to define the NDCS. He preferred to refer to the drug problem as a malignancy.[10] During his tenure, McCaffrey did advocate for treatment, but the ONDCP budget remained distributed two-thirds supply reduction, one-third prevention and treatment. McCaffrey also was the ONDCP director during the Plan Colombia initiative of 1999, a $1.3 billion effort to eradicate coca cultivation in Colombia (cocaine is produced from coca leaves), an effort that has continued in the Bush administration. Following George W. Bush's election in 2000, John Walters was confirmed as ONDCP director in 2001. He continues to serve as this is written (June 2006). Walters first worked at ONDCP from 1986 to 1993. He was chief of staff for Drug Czar William Bennett and Deputy Director for Supply Reduction from 1991 to 1993. During Walters' tenure, ONDCP has fiercely battled efforts by states to liberalize marijuana laws (i.e., medical marijuana laws, reductions in criminal penalties for possession) and has implemented the President's Access to Recovery initiative, a $100 million per year program to increase treatment and recovery options for alcoholics and drug addicts. Under Walters' direction, an increasing percentage of NDCS resources have been allocated to efforts to reduce the amount of illegal drugs from entering the country compared to funding for prevention and treatment.

Goals of the War on Drugs: Supply and Demand Reduction

As was discussed in the previous sections, the priorities of ONDCP have been defined by Congress. ONDCP has been charged with decreasing the availability of drugs in the United States. That is called "supply reduction." Furthermore, ONDCP is responsible for preventing the use of illicit drugs by young people (prevention) and for reducing the number of users (treatment). Together, prevention and treatment are called "demand reduction."

You may have noticed that our legal drugs, tobacco, and alcohol are not the focus of ONDCP's mandate. There will be much more to say about this in later chapters of this book. At this point, it should be noted that tobacco use has been the focus of federal initiatives. They just aren't in the scope of responsibility of ONDCP. The prevention of underage drinking has been included in some ONDCP initiatives. However, the amount of money dedicated to the prevention of underage drinking is minimal compared to other activities. Again, there will be a great deal of attention directed to this issue in later chapters.

Supply reduction is divided into three parts: domestic law enforcement, interdiction, and international. Domestic law enforcement involves all of the activities to stop the production and distribution of illicit drugs in the United States. Most people are familiar with the DEA and have seen media depictions of drug busts by DEA agents. This would be considered domestic law enforcement. Interdiction includes all efforts to stop illegal drugs from entering the United States. Checking cars at the U.S./Mexican border, U.S. Coast Guard intercepts of boats carrying drugs, and Customs inspections are examples of interdiction. International efforts include spraying coca leaves and poppy fields (used to produce heroin) in foreign countries and working with foreign governments to disrupt drug cartels.

As stated earlier, demand reduction involves prevention and treatment. Generally, prevention efforts involve activities designed to stop young people from using illicit drugs or to intervene in the progression of experimental use of these substances to regular use. Treatment includes services for people who have already developed problems with illicit drugs. Prevention and treatment research is also included in the demand reduction portion of the NDCS.

Table 1.1 displays the NDCS budgets from 1996 through 2005. The Bush administration changed accounting procedures for the NDCS budget in 2002 so that only activities strongly associated with the NDCS would be considered part of the NDCS budget. This resulted in a significant decrease in the supply reduction budget from 2001 to 2002. As can be seen, more than two-thirds of the NDCS budget was dedicated to supply reduction until the accounting changes of 2002. Since 2002, the percentage of total NDCS dollars allocated to supply reduction has been increasing compared to demand reduction. President Bush's 2006 budget continued the trend toward increasing the supply reduction budget at the expense of the demand reduction budget. In 2006, 62 percent of the budget is allocated to supply reduction.[11] The enhancement to supply reduction is in domestic law enforcement.

Over the last 10 years (1996–2005), the United States has spent nearly $94 billion to reduce the supply of illegal drugs in this country and almost $51 billion to reduce the demand for illicit drugs.

Do We Need to Spend Billions?

It may seem obvious that drug abuse is a major societal problem that requires a huge financial commitment by the federal government. However, it is instructive to examine the data on the estimated costs of drug abuse to our country to quantify the scope of the problem. ONDCP commissioned a study on the economic costs of drug abuse in the United States from 1992 to 2002.[12] The estimated cost of drug abuse in 2002 was nearly $181 billion. Of that amount, nearly 60 percent involved crime-related costs, including productivity losses due to incarceration and crime careers; local, state, and federal corrections; police protection; legal adjudication; and the NDCS supply reduction expenditures. The remaining 40 percent involved healthcare costs (approximately 8 percent) and productivity losses due to premature death and drug abuse related illnesses (approximately 32 percent). According to this study, there were an estimated 23,500 drug-related deaths in 2000. These deaths were caused by overdose, poisoning, homicide, AIDS, and hepatitis.[13]

Table 1.1
NDCS Budgets 1996–2005 (dollar figures in billions)

	1996 $	%	1997 $	%	1998 $	%	1999 $	%	2000 $	%	2001 $	%	2002 $	%	2003 $	%	2004 $	%	2005 $	%	Total $
Supply reduction	9.01	67	10.09	67	10.63	66	12.40	70	12.92	72	12.18	67	5.87	56	6.27	57	6.88	58	7.64	60	93.89
Domestic law enforcement	7.40	55	7.95	53	8.53	53	NA	NA	NA	NA	9.46	52	2.87	27	3.02	27	3.19	27	3.32	26	NA
International	0.29	2	0.42	3	0.48	3	NA	NA	NA	NA	0.66	4	1.08	10	1.11	10	1.16	10	1.39	11	NA
Interdiction	1.32	10	1.72	11	1.61	10	NA	NA	NA	NA	2.05	11	1.91	18	2.15	19	2.53	21	2.93	23	NA
Demand reduction	4.44	33	4.94	33	5.47	34	5.31	30	5.02	28	5.91	33	4.78	45	4.81	43	4.99	42	5.01	40	50.68
Prevention	1.61	12	1.87	12	2.25	14	1.95	11	2.15	12	2.58	14	2.00	19	1.94	17	1.96	17	1.95	15	20.26
Treatment	2.83	21	3.07	21	3.22	20	3.36	19	2.87	16	3.34	18	2.78	26	2.88	25	3.03	26	3.05	24	30.43
Total	13.45		15.03		16.10		17.71		17.94		18.10		10.65		11.08		11.87		12.64		144.57

Notes: In 1999 and 2000, the NDCS reported budget breakdowns by goal rather than by function. Therefore, the supply reduction subcategories could not be calculated and the demand reduction subcategories may not be exact. All budget figures are final budget figures. The subcategory percentages and dollar figures may not add up exactly to the supply reduction and demand reduction categories because of rounding.
Sources: Office of National Drug Control Policy, National Drug Control Strategies, 1996–2005. References to each separate document are in the "Notes," Chapter 2.

As has been stated, the mission of ONDCP does not involve alcohol abuse. However, in order to gain a perspective on the scope of the drug problem, it is helpful to compare the costs to our country as a result of alcohol abuse to those that result from illegal drug abuse. Unfortunately, the last study of the costs of alcohol abuse was in 1998. So some extrapolations will have to be made in order to compare the costs of alcohol abuse in 1998 and the costs of illegal drug abuse in 2002. In 1998, the economic costs of alcohol abuse in the United States was estimated to be $184.6 billion[14] (in 1998, the economic costs of drug abuse were estimated to be $99.3 billion).[15] The crime-related portion of this total was $16.4 billion or nearly 9 percent with the remainder in health care expenditures ($26.3 billion, 14 percent), lost productivity unrelated to crime ($124.1 billion, 67 percent), motor vehicle accidents ($15.7 billion, 9 percent), and other impacts on society ($2 billion, 1 percent). More than 100,000 deaths per year are related to alcohol abuse (traffic accidents, homicide, suicide, cirrhosis of the liver).[16]

In Table 1.2, the economic costs of alcohol abuse in 2002 were computed by assuming that the same relationship between the economic costs of alcohol abuse and drug abuse in 1998 continue to exist in 2002.

As can be seen, the economic costs of alcohol abuse are nearly double those of drug abuse and more than four times as many people die each year from alcohol abuse than from drug abuse. Due to the fact that most of the abuse of drugs results from substances that are illegal, most of the costs of drug abuse are crime-related. Two-thirds of the economic costs of alcohol abuse are related to lost productivity. All of this certainly raises the question of whether ONDCP's focus on illicit drugs is misguided. To be fair, the money in the NDCS budget devoted to treatment does support programs that provide services for alcoholics as well as other drug addicts and other programs targeting alcohol abuse and underage drinking have been implemented. However, in spite of the evidence that alcohol abuse is far more damaging to our country than drug abuse, far more federal resources are devoted to issues involving illegal drugs than to alcohol.

This is not to argue that the problems caused by drug abuse are trivial and should not be the focus of federal initiatives designed to reduce these problems. A problem that results in over 20,000 deaths annually and has associated economic costs of nearly $200 billion is clearly not trivial. The comparison of drug abuse to alcohol abuse was made to illustrate that both of these problems are worthy of attention. However, the general public tends to separate these two issues, mainly because alcohol is legal and most of the drugs discussed here are not. Furthermore, illicit drug issues are dramatically depicted in news stories and in entertainment media. Drug busts, injecting heroin, and smoking crack make compelling television and movie stories. In our culture, there is a tendency to view alcohol abuse resulting in intoxication as humorous while the use of most illicit drugs as sinister. And,

Table 1.2
Comparison of Costs of Alcohol Abuse and Drug Abuse (dollar figures in billions)

	Total costs	Crime related	Health care	Productivity loss	Motor vehicle	Other	Annual deaths
Alcohol abuse	$336.3	$30.3	$47.1	$225.3	$30.3	$3.3	100,000
Drug abuse	$180.9	$107.8	$15.7	$60.1	NA	NA	23,500

Sources: Office of National Drug Control Policy 2004; Harwood 2000; National Institute on Alcohol Abuse and Alcoholism 1996.

our NDCS contributes to the perception that illicit drug problems are different than alcohol problems by the focus on illicit drugs. This issue will be discussed in much greater detail in later chapters of this book.

Conclusion

For the past 10 years, the United States has spent approximately $145 billion to reduce the supply of illicit drugs in this country and to reduce the demand for these substances through prevention and treatment. There are data that would suggest that this money has not produced the desired results.

Given the tremendous amount of financial resources devoted to this problem and the fact that there does not seem to be progress, it is disconcerting that federal officials are resistant to considering alternatives to our NDCS. There have been prohibitions against discussing controversial issues such as harm reduction, decriminalization, and legalization of illicit drugs. Furthermore, the NDCS has not focused on alcohol abuse, a problem that causes far more harm than drug abuse.

Regardless of priorities, the fact remains that the federal government allocates billions of dollars each year to the goals of supply and demand reduction of illicit drugs. It is time to examine the specific activities that this money has supported and the outcomes that have been produced.

Two

The National Drug Control Strategy, 1996–2005

Introduction

Each NDCS report contains a series of activities designed to implement the strategy. Although there are always new initiatives in each strategy, there are also core activities that are funded every year. For example, in each NDCS budget, there is funding for the Department of Defense and the State Department to conduct various activities related to international efforts and interdiction. This involves crop eradication in source countries like Colombia, assisting governments such as Mexico with combating drug producers and traffickers, and disrupting money laundering operations around the world. In the more recent budgets, the Department of Homeland Security has a sizeable budget because it is responsible for Customs and Border Protection, Immigration and Customs Enforcement, and the U.S. Coast Guard. As might be expected, the activities of these agencies involve protecting the borders of the United States from the influx of illicit drugs. In addition, the Justice Department receives funding for the DEA, the Interagency Crime and Drug Enforcement, and the Office of Justice Programs. These agencies are involved with disrupting drug production, drug distribution, and money laundering in the United States and elsewhere. The range of activities of all of these agencies involved with supply reduction is immense, as it should be with a combined budget in 2005 of over $7 billion for the agencies mentioned.

One interesting initiative that has been funded for more than 10 years is the High Intensity Drug Trafficking Area (HIDTA) program, a part of ONDCP. In the 1996 NDCS, there is an entire chapter devoted to HIDTA. HIDTA regions in the United States were designated based on the extent to which an area was a center of illegal drug production, manufacturing, importation, or distribution. HIDTA funding was designed to reduce drug trafficking in the designated area and includes local, state, and federal joint ventures involving interdiction, investigation, prosecution, treatment, and prevention.[1] HIDTA funding went from $103 million in 1996 to over $226 million in 2005.[2] However, in recommending a dramatic reduction in the HIDTA program for fiscal year 2006, the 2005 NDCS reported that "The ... assessment finds that the HIDTA program has not been able to demonstrate results."[3]

In the demand reduction area, the vast majority of funding is in the Department of Health and Human Services. In 2005, about one-third of that money went to the National Institute on Drug Abuse to conduct research on pharmacology, drug abuse, drug treatment and prevention, and related topics. The remaining two-thirds were directed to the Substance Abuse and Mental Health Services Administration (SAMHSA). In 2005, nearly three-quarters of the SAMHSA budget was allocated to the Substance Abuse Prevention and Treatment Block Grant (Block Grant), which funds public-sector alcohol and other drug treatment programs in all 50 states. This provides treatment services for people who cannot afford it. In addition, 20 percent of the Block Grant money is set aside for prevention programs.

Demand reduction funding is also allocated to the Veterans Health Administration to provide treatment services for veterans and the Department of Education for the Safe and Drug-Free Schools and Communities program. Most of the Safe and Drug-Free Schools and Communities money is distributed to state and local school districts for drug and violence prevention programs. It should be noted that the 2005 NDCS recommended, "... to terminate funding for the state grants portion of the Safe and Drug-Free Schools and Communities program because of its inability to demonstrate effectiveness and the fact that grant funds are spread too thinly to support quality interventions."[4]

Some of the specific NDCS activities from each year from 1996 to 2005 will now be discussed. Activities in each NDCS are proposed for the following fiscal year. For example, the activities mentioned in the 1996 NDCS were implemented in the 1997 fiscal year.

1996[5]

Since this is the first NDCS discussed in this book, some of the 1996 activities mentioned are from the previous years in the Clinton administration.

Supply Reduction: A major focus of the supply reduction effort was the Southwest border region. An additional 657 Customs staff were budgeted for the Southwest border. In addition, the Immigration and Naturalization Service received an additional 105 Border Patrol agents to reduce the flow of illegal drugs across the Southwest border. Finally, the Department of Justice initiated the Southwest Border Project to target drug trafficking organizations in this region by disrupting their operations and striving to dismantle their infrastructures.

In 1995, President Clinton shifted the emphasis in interdiction from drug transit areas to source production countries. In other words, rather than targeting the places where illegal drugs are transported for entry into the United States, the focus shifted to actual countries that produced drugs (e.g., coca production in Central America). This shift was reflected in the proposed 1997 budget by increasing international narcotics control by nearly 43 percent. The activities included eradication, alternative crop development programs, interdiction efforts, and initiatives to dismantle foreign drug trafficking organizations. Domestically, there was continued funding for the DEA's Domestic Cannabis Eradication/Suppression Program, which provides resources for state and local law enforcement agencies to destroy marijuana plants and arrest cultivators, and a program to curb marijuana growing on public lands.

Domestic law enforcement was also a priority area. President Clinton had a major initiative to put more police on the streets and included this as part of the NDCS. This program was called Community Oriented Policing (COPS). The DEA received funding for Mobile Enforcement Teams to assist state and local law enforcement with disrupting and dismantling drug trafficking gangs. The HIDTA program, with six HIDTAs funded by 1997, has already been mentioned. Finally, a drug testing program for arrestees was implemented.

Demand Reduction: In the prevention area, the Safe and Drug-Free Schools and Communities Program, that provided grants to state educational agencies (and then to local school districts) for drug and violence prevention, has already been mentioned. During the Clinton administration, the Community Partnership Projects were started. This program was designed to assist community coalitions with developing and maintaining long-term prevention strategies. In addition, the Corporation for National and Community Service received funds to expand a volunteer program and the Department of Labor Drug Prevention Programs were funded to assist at-risk youth to acquire skills to succeed at work and to avoid drugs.

In the treatment area, money was provided for grants to start Drug Courts (court-mandated treatment and related services for nonviolent offenders) and for funding for substance abuse treatment in state and federal prisons. These programs were in addition to the Block Grant and Veterans Administration funding for treatment mentioned earlier.

1997[6]

Supply Reduction: The Immigration and Naturalization Service received additional funds to implement the Southwest Border Project by hiring more Border Patrol agents. More money was also provided to the State Department's International Narcotics and Law Enforcement Affairs to increase their activities in Peru. President Clinton's effort to increase the number of police officers was emphasized by an increase in the funding devoted to the COPS program.

Demand Reduction: In the treatment area, more money was devoted to Drug Courts and a Youth Treatment Initiative was started. The Youth Treatment Initiative was to support interventions for juvenile offenders. More money was also allocated to the National Institute on Drug Abuse to conduct research.

The major demand reduction initiatives in the 1997 NDCS involved prevention. Congress passed H.R. 956, the Drug-Free Communities Act of 1997. This Act authorized grants for community coalitions to develop and implement comprehensive, long-term plans and programs to prevent and treat substance abuse among youth. The program was to be administered by ONDCP and it continues today. In addition, the Safe and Drug-Free Schools program received an 11.5 percent increase to $620 million.

The highlight of the prevention initiatives was the Secretary of Health and Human Services' 5-year Youth Substance Abuse Prevention Initiative (YSAPI). The primary purpose of YSAPI was to reduce marijuana use by youth. A total of $175 million was allocated for a national media campaign and $98 million for other activities, including State Incentive Grants (SIGs). States could apply for funding of $3 million a year for 3 years to promote the implementation of model prevention programs (programs with demonstrated effectiveness) in communities. Over the 5-year YSAPI period, nearly every state received a SIG.

1998[7]

Supply Reduction: A major new initiative involved the Andean Ridge region. A large increase in the budgets for the Defense and State Departments was provided for coca eradication, alternative crop development programs, and other counterdrug activities. These funds would be greatly expanded by more than $800 million in supplemental funding in the 1999 fiscal year. The Coast Guard received additional money for capital improvements to enhance interdiction capabilities in the Caribbean. The Treasury Department was allocated additional funds for nonintrusive inspection techniques (e.g., mobile and fixed X-ray systems) along the Southwest border. The Border Patrol in the Immigration and Naturalization Service received money for additional agents and deployment of the Integrated Surveillance Intelligence System and Remote Video Surveillance equipment. This system used infrared and color cameras with ground sensors. New methamphetamine and heroin initiatives were funded through the DEA. This money provided the DEA with 378 new positions, including 200 special agents, to combat methamphetamine and heroin trafficking, production, and distribution.

Demand Reduction: The capacity of states to provide treatment was enhanced by a $200 million increase in the Block Grant. The National Institute on Drug Abuse received additional money for research on drug addiction. A new Drug Intervention Program was funded through the Office of Justice Programs to implement drug testing, treatment, and graduated sanctions for drug offenders. Funding for the Drug-Free Communities Act was doubled and additional funding was provided to the Department of Education to fund 1,300 school drug prevention coordinators.

1999[8]

Supply Reduction: In addition to the more than $800 million in supplemental funding for coca eradication and other counterdrug operations in the Andean Region, more money was allocated to the Bureau of International Narcotics and Law Enforcement Affairs for operations in the Andean countries and Mexico. The Immigration and Naturalization Service needed more money to deploy the Integrated Surveillance Information System and the DEA received additional funding to implement an office automation system called FIREBIRD. The Department of Defense was allocated funding to develop Forward Operating Locations to support transit and source zone air operations.

Demand Reduction: The Drug Intervention Program mentioned in 1998 received additional funding. Increased funds to hire more school coordinators were also provided. The National Youth Anti-Drug Media Campaign (part of YSAPI) received an increase of $10 million to $195 million and the Block Grant was also increased. A new treatment initiative was created called "Targeted Capacity Expansion Grants." These grants expanded treatment in areas of existing or emerging need, such as specialized treatment for women and adolescents.

2000[9]

Supply Reduction: In fiscal year 2000 and fiscal year 2001, a combined $1.6 billion was allocated for counterdrug efforts in Colombia. This was a part of Plan Colombia, a project to address the drug and related social and economic issues in this country. The funding was for counterdrug regional interdiction and alternative crop development and was designed to prevent cocaine traffickers from moving operations from Peru and Bolivia to Colombia. In addition, more money was allocated for the DEA's FIREBIRD automated system, the Department of Defense's Forward Operating Locations in Ecuador, Aruba, and Curacao, an additional 430 Border Patrol agents, and continued deployment of the Integrated Surveillance Information System. It should be noted that the Integrated Surveillance Intelligence System is not highlighted in any further NDCS reports. However, according to a report in the *Washington Post*, the system has been plagued by defective equipment, poor installation, and overcharging by the contractor.[10] The Coast Guard received additional money to support drug interdiction efforts in the Caribbean and Eastern Pacific. Due to increased prosecution of drug cases, $420 million was allocated for prison construction.

Demand Reduction: The Drug Intervention Program (see 1998) was restructured and provided with $100 million. Drug Courts and Residential Substance Abuse Treatment (intensive treatment for chronic addicts) received small increases in funding. ONDCP continued funding the National Youth Anti-Drug Media Campaign at $195 million but also announced a $2 billion, multiyear national media campaign. The Safe and Drug-Free Schools and Communities program received an additional $50 million to support communitywide prevention activities and to continue the School Coordinator Initiative from 1998. The Block Grant, Targeted Capacity Expansion, and research all received some increase in funding. The funding for the Drug-Free Communities Act was increased to $35 million.

2001

Since this was the first year of the Bush administration, there was no NDCS for 2001. An annual report was prepared by General McCaffrey, the director of ONDCP in the Clinton administration

2002[11]

Supply Reduction: The first Bush administration NDCS included an increase of over $100 million for the Andean Counterdrug Initiative and money for more border agents.

Demand Reduction: There were budget increases in the Block Grant, Targeted Capacity Expansion grants, Residential Substance Abuse Treatment program, Drug Courts, and the Drug-Free Communities Act Program. A new initiative was the Parents Drug Corps Program, a $5 million program funded through the Corporation for National and Community Service to train parents in drug prevention skills and methods.

2003[12]

Supply Reduction: The Organized Crime Drug Enforcement Task Forces (OCDETF) Program in the Department of Justice was restructured and new initiatives were proposed. This included 192 positions for the Consolidated Priority Organization Target (CPOT) List Initiative, "... to generate and advance investigations of command and control targets linked to the Attorney General's CPOT list"[13] (a list of major drug trafficking and money laundering organizations); the Automated Tracking Initiative to scan, analyze, and disseminate drug investigation information to OCDETF agencies; and the Financial and Money Laundering Initiative, including 83 positions to expand OCDETF financial and money laundering investigations. Three hundred twenty-nine positions were added to the DEA for the CPOT List Initiative. The Department of Defense was given an additional $25 million to expand support for the counterdrug activities in Colombia.

Demand Reduction: The National Youth Anti-Drug Media Campaign was cut to $170 million. In addition, a new strategy was adopted requiring testing of all TV ads for effectiveness, shift of the target audience to ages 14–16, modifying advertisement to focus primarily on marijuana, more oversight by ONDCP, and a harder-hitting advertisement style. The Drug-Free Communities Act program was increased to $70 million. In the 2003 NDCS, the Safe and Drug-Free Schools and Communities was described as ineffective. However, $584 million was allocated to the program, including $8 million in grants for drug testing programs in schools.

You may recall that the YSAPI program described in the 1997 NDCS included the SIG, awards to states to help communities implement model prevention programs. Nearly every state received about $9 million over 3 years to implement the state SIG. In 2003, a new prevention initiative was proposed, the Strategic Prevention Framework State Incentive Grants (SPF SIG). Beginning in fiscal year 2004, 19 states and 2 jurisdictions received $230 million over 5 years to implement the SPF SIG. In contrast to the original SIG program, the SPF SIG program requires states to form epidemiology workgroups and utilize a prevention planning process to determine needs and appropriate prevention strategies.

The highlight of the demand reduction NDCS was the President's Access to Recovery Initiative. This is a voucher system in which those in need of treatment or recovery services could choose the provider that best meets their needs. The intent of this initiative was to increase the involvement of faith-based organizations in providing treatment and recovery services. The President requested $600 million over 3 years for Access to Recovery but Congress has cut this request in half for the last 2 years. Increases in Drug Courts and research for the National Institute on Drug Abuse were also included in the NDCS.

2004[14]

Supply Reduction: The CPOT List Initiative and the various other OCDETF initiatives were allocated more money. In addition, the Immigration and Customs Enforcement was provided with an additional $28 million to increase the flight hours of P-3 aircraft, designed to provide radar coverage in mountains, jungles, and over large bodies of water.

Demand Reduction: An additional $23 million was allocated for student drug testing grants and the Drug-Free Communities Act Programs received an additional $10.4 million. (The program began at $10 million and was now at $80 million per year.) Drug Courts and the National Institute on Drug Abuse (research) also received funding increases.

2005[15]

Supply Reduction: As in 2004, more money was allocated for the CPOT List Initiative and various OCDETF initiatives. In addition, an additional $22 million was requested for DEA Central/Southwest Asian Operations to support poppy investigations and enforcement in Afghanistan. The Department of State also asked for an additional $166.2 million for counternarcotics programs in Afghanistan.

Demand Reduction: The President requested more money for the Access to Recovery Program. However, Congress maintained the program at current funding levels. An additional $30.6 million was requested for Drug Courts and a small amount ($5.8 million) was allocated for grants to support screening and brief interventions, programs intended to intervene with nondependent drug users before they progress to abuse or dependence. An additional $15.4 million was requested for student drug testing programs. Finally, the 2005 NDCS did recommend termination of the Safe and Drug-Free Schools and Communities program and replacing this program with grants to local school districts to implement research-based programs. However, Congress did not enact this recommendation.

Performance Indicators

After spending nearly $145 billion over the last 10 years, it is certainly reasonable to expect that the NDCS activities have resulted in positive changes. Logically, it would be expected that each NDCS would include performance indicators and some type of data to show progress or the lack thereof. In fact, the ONDCP Reauthorization Act of 1998 did include five specific targets to be achieved by the end of 2003.[16] Furthermore, the Act stipulates that the ONDCP director establish additional targets to be achieved in future years.[17] All targets involve reductions in drug use, reductions in drug availability, and reductions in the consequences of drug abuse. The 1999 NDCS, developed during the Clinton administration, contained 12 such targets, using a base year of 1996 and goals for 2002 and 2007.[18] Ironically, there is no mention of any progress measures for these targets in the 2000 NDCS or subsequent NDCS reports in the Bush administration. However, in the 2002 NDCS, the Bush administration did establish 2-year and 5-year goals[19]:

2-year goals	A 10 percent reduction in current use of illegal drugs by the 12–17 age group
	A 10 percent reduction in current use of illegal drugs by adults age 18 and older
5-year goals	A 25 percent reduction in current use of illegal drugs by the 12–17 age group
	A 25 percent reduction in current use of illegal drugs by adults age 18 and older

The baseline year for these goals was 2000. The Bush administration NDCS reports do not mention the five targets included in the ONDCP Reauthorization Act of 1998. It is certainly surprising that more goals relating to more aspects of the NDCS were not specified in the Bush administration NDCS plans, given the billions of dollars being spent to implement the NDCS.

The fairest approach to measure the effectiveness of the NDCS seems to be to examine all of the targets or goals in the Clinton and Bush NDCS reports. These targets and goals have been grouped by their relationship to substance use, drug availability, or the consequences of drug abuse.

The detailed information regarding each of the targets and goals in this section is summarized in Table 2.1.

Most of the data relevant to these targets and goals have come from tables and charts in the NDCS reports. For some targets, there are no direct performance measures. In these cases, an attempt has been made to find some information related to the target. Another issue involves the surveys used as performance measures for some targets. For example, the goals in the 2002 NDCS specified that the National Household Survey on Drug Abuse (retitled "National Household Survey on Drug Use and Health" after the 2002 NDCS was released) would be used as the performance measure, with 2000 data as the baseline. However, the survey procedures were changed in 2002 and, therefore, comparisons between 2000 and 2002 cannot be made. This same survey is referenced as a performance measure in the first of the five Congressional mandated targets from the ONDCP Reauthorization Act of 1998. Due to the changes in the National Household

Table 2.1
Summary of NDCS Targets

Targets	Indicators	Results
I. Substance Use Targets and Goals		
A. Reduce the overall prevalence of illicit drug use by 25% by 2002 and by 50% by 2007	Tables 2.2 and 2.3	Not achieved
B. Reduce the prevalence of illicit drug and alcohol use among youth by 20% by 2002 and 50% by 2007. Reduce the prevalence of tobacco consumption among youth by 25% by 2002 and 55% by 2007	Tables 2.2, 2.3, 2.4, 2.5, 2.6, and 2.7	2002 illicit drug use and alcohol target achieved for 8th graders. 2002 and 2007 tobacco use targets achieved for 8th and 10th graders. No other targets achieved for 8th, 10th, and 12th graders or for combined grades
C. Increase the average age of first-time drug use by 12 months by 2002 and 36 months by 2007	Table 2.9, Youth Risk Behavior Surveillance Survey	Not achieved
D. Reduce the prevalence of drug use in the workplace by 25% by 2002 and 50% by 2007	Table 2.10	Not achieved
E. Reduce the number of chronic drug users by 20% by 2002 and 50% by 2007	National Household Survey	No evidence to support progress
F. 10% reduction in current use of illegal drugs by 12–17 age group from 2000 to 2002	Tables 2.2, 2.3, 2.4, and 2.5	Target achieved for 8th graders but not for 10th or 12th graders or combined grades
G. 10% reduction in current use of illegal drugs by adults age 18 and older from 2000 to 2002	Tables 2.2, 2.3, 2.4, and 2.5	Not achieved
H. 25% reduction in current use of illegal drugs by 12–17 age group from 2000 to 2005	Tables 2.2, 2.3, 2.4, and 2.5	Target achieved for 8th graders but not for 10th or 12th graders or combined grades

I. 25% reduction in current use of illegal drugs by adults age 18 and older from 2000 to 2005	Tables 2.2, 2.3, 2.4, and 2.5	Not achieved
J. Reduction of unlawful drug use to 3% or less of the U.S. population by December 31, 2003 (as measured in terms of overall illicit drug use during the past 30 days by National Household Survey on Drug Abuse (NHSDA)) and achievement of at least 20% of such reduction during 1999, 2000, 2001, 2002, and 2003, respectively	Table 2.2	Not achieved
K. Reduction of unlawful adolescent drug use (as measured in terms of illicit drug use during the past 30 days by the Monitoring the Future (MTF) study of the University of Michigan or the National PRIDE survey conducted by the Parents' Resource Institute for Drug Education) to 3% or less of the U.S. adolescent population by December 31, 2003, and achievement of at least 20% of such reduction during 1999, 2000, 2001, 2002, and 2003, respectively	Table 2.3, PRIDE Survey	Not achieved
2. Supply Reduction Targets and Goals		
A. Reduce the domestic availability of illegal drugs by 25% in 2002 and 50% by 2007	Tables 2.11 and 2.12, National Drug Threat Assessment	Not achieved

(continued)

21

Table 2.1
(continued)

Targets	Indicators	Results
B. Reduce the rate of shipment of illegal drugs from source countries by 15% by 2002 and 30% by 2007	Tables 2.11 and 2.12, National Drug Threat Assessment	Not achieved
C. Reduce the rate at which illegal drugs enter the United States by 10% by 2002 and 20% by 2007	Tables 2.11 and 2.12, National Drug Threat Assessment	Not achieved
D. Reduce the production of methamphetamine and cultivation of marijuana in the United States by 20% by 2002 and 50% by 2007	Tables 2.11 and 2.12, National Drug Threat Assessment	Not achieved
E. Reduce trafficker success rate in the United States	Tables 2.11 and 2.12, National Drug Threat Assessment	Not achieved
F. Reduction of cocaine, heroin, marijuana, and methamphetamine availability in the United States by 80% by December 31, 2003	National Drug Threat Assessment	Not achieved
G. Reduction of nationwide average street purity levels for cocaine, heroin, marijuana, and methamphetamine (as estimated by the interagency drug-flow assessment process, the Drug Enforcement Administration, and other national drug-control program agencies) by 60%	Table 2.12	Not achieved

60% by December 31, 2003, and achievement of at least 20% of such reduction during 1999, 2000, 2001, 2002, and 2003, respectively		
3. Targets and Goals Related to the Consequences of Drug Abuse		
A. Reduce crime associated with drug trafficking and use by 15% by 2002 and 30% by 2007	Table 2.13, Arrestee Drug Abuse Monitoring Program	Not achieved
B. Reduce the health and social costs associated with drug trafficking and use by 10% by 2002 and 25% by 2007	Table 2.14, "Economic Costs of Drug Abuse in the United States: 1992–2002,' deaths from drug use, injecting drug users with AIDS, drug-related emergency room visits, tuberculosis among injecting drug users, Youth Risk Behavior Surveillance Survey, school drop-out rate	Tuberculosis decreased among injecting drug users. Decreases in some youth risk behaviors. No other data to support target
C. Reduction of drug-related crime in the United States by 50% by December 31, 2003, and achievement of at least 20% of such reduction during 1999, 2000, 2001, 2002, and 2003	Crime-related costs of drug abuse, number of incarcerated drug offenders, Arrestee Drug Abuse Monitoring Program	No data to support achievement of target

Survey on Drug Use and Health,[20] other surveys will be used as performance measures and the results of the National Household Survey will only be used to illustrate certain points.

Substance Use Targets and Goals

Substance use targets from the Clinton administration 1999 NDCS: These targets all use a base year of 1996. Unless otherwise noted, all data in the tables are reported as percentages.

Target 1. Reduce the overall prevalence of illicit drug use by 25 percent by 2002 and 50 percent by 2007.

It is common to look at 30-day prevalence as the metric for "use" and that is the standard in the NDCS. This means that people are asked if they have used a particular substance at any time in the last 30 days.

The major problem with gathering data directly related to this target involves the changes in the National Household Survey. This is the only major federally sponsored survey that examines tobacco, alcohol, and other drug use among adults. The process to collect data involves interviews with participants. As previously stated, the changes in survey procedures do not allow for long-range comparisons. Survey procedures were changed in 1999 and again in 2002. For example, in 1999, computer-assisted interviewing was substituted for paper-and-pencil data collection. In 2002, participants received an incentive payment for participation and quality control procedures were implemented for data collection. While these changes may not seem to be dramatic, the published results contain cautions to avoid comparisons between years that utilized different survey procedures. Therefore, for our purposes, the data from 1996 to 1998 can be compared; the data from 1999 to 2001 can be compared; and the data from 2002 to 2004 can be compared. As of June 2006, the 2005 data had not been released. In 2004, 67,760 people representing all 50 states were interviewed.

Table 2.2 displays this information for all surveyed participants, aged 12 and older and for 12- to 17-year-olds (the data for 12- to 17-year-olds will be discussed in Target 2). Although a 10-year comparison cannot be made, it is difficult to find any support for a reduction in the overall prevalence of illicit drug use by 25 percent from 1996 to 2002, or 2004 for that matter. From 1996 to 1998, there was virtually no change. From 1999 to 2001, prevalence went up. From 2002 to 2004, there was a reduction of 4.8 percent.

Because of the changes in the National Household Survey, most attention has been directed to the annual Monitoring the Future Study sponsored by the National Institute on Drug Abuse. The primary purpose of this survey is to

Table 2.2
Illicit Drug Use in Past Month,
National Household Survey

	12 and Older	12–17
1996	6.1	9.0
1997	6.4	11.4
1998	6.2	9.9
1999	6.3	9.8
2000	6.3	9.8
2001	7.1	10.8
2002	8.3	11.6
2003	8.2	11.2
2004	7.9	10.6

Source: Office of Applied Studies, Substance Abuse and Mental Health Services Administration. 2005. National Survey on Drug Use and Health. http://oas.samhsa.gov/nsduh.htm#N5DUHinfo.

examine tobacco, alcohol, and other drug use among 8th, 10th, and 12th grade students. However, the survey also collects follow-up data from college students and young adults (ages 19–28). In contrast to the interview format of the National Household Survey, questionnaires are completed by participants in the Monitoring the Future Survey. For example, 49,500 students in 406 secondary schools were sampled in 2004. Each year, an effort is made to resurvey 1,200 former high school seniors for the college student and young adult samples. The results of this survey from 1996 to 2005, for any illicit drug use (i.e., the student reported using any illicit drug in the past 30 days), are displayed in Table 2.3. Among 8th graders, the target was met for 2002 and appears to be achievable by 2007. The 2002 goal was not achieved by any other age group, although 10th graders achieved a 25 percent reduction by 2005. It is noticeable that 12th graders, college students, and young adults all showed increased illicit drug use from 1996 to 2002 and this trend continued for college students and young adults through 2004 (as of June 2006, the 2005 data for college students and young adults were not available). Twelfth graders showed some decrease by 2005. (The column "8th–12th" will be discussed under Target 2. The two final rows of this table relate to the Bush goals in the 2002 NDCS and will be discussed later in this chapter.)

Obviously, there is no evidence that Target 1 had been achieved by 2002 or that the 2007 goal is likely to be met. On the contrary, among college students and young adults the trend reflected increased illicit drug use.

Table 2.3
30-Day Prevalence of Any Illicit Drugs, Monitoring the Future

	8th Grade	10th Grade	12th Grade	8th–12th Grades	College Students	Young Adults
1996	14.6	23.2	24.6	20.8	17.6	15.8
1997	12.9	23.0	26.2	20.7	19.2	16.4
1998	12.1	21.5	25.6	19.7	19.7	16.1
1999	12.2	22.1	25.9	20.1	21.6	17.1
2000	11.9	22.5	24.9	19.8	21.5	18.1
2001	11.7	22.7	25.7	20.0	21.9	18.8
2002	10.4	20.8	25.4	18.9	21.5	18.9
2003	9.7	19.5	24.1	17.8	21.4	19.9
2004	8.4	18.3	23.4	16.7	21.2	19.1
2005	8.5	17.3	23.1	16.3	NA	NA
1996–2002	−28.8%	−10.3%	+3.3%	−9.1	+22.2%	+19.6%
1996–end	−41.8%	−25.4%	−6.1%	−21.6	+20.1%	+20.9%
2000–2002	−12.6%	−7.6%	+2.0%	−4.5	0%	+4.0%
2000–end	−28.6%	−23.1%	−7.2%	−17.7	−1.4%	+5.5%

Note: "End" refers to 2005 for 8th, 10th, and 12th graders and 2004 for college students and young adults.
Source: Johnston, L. D., P. M. O'Malley, J. G. Bachman, and J. E. Schulenberg. 2005. *Monitoring the Future National Results on Adolescent Drug Use: Overview of Key Findings, 2004*. NIH Publication No. 05–5726. Bethesda, MD: National Institute on Drug Abuse.

Target 2. Reduce the prevalence of illicit drug and alcohol use among youth by 20 percent by 2002 and 50 percent by 2007. Reduce the prevalence of tobacco consumption among youth by 25 percent by 2002 and 55 percent by 2007.

The first part of this target has been discussed in Target 1. The Monitoring the Future Survey data in Table 2.3 shows that the target was achieved only for 8th graders for the 2002 goal, although the trend was in the right direction for 10th graders. Unfortunately, this survey does not report a compiled category for 8th, 10th, and 12th graders. However, an average of the three percentages can be computed.[21] Looking at these data, it can be seen that the 2002 target was not achieved nor is the 2007 target likely to be achieved. Furthermore, the data from the National Household Survey in Table 2.2 does not provide evidence to support the goal for 2002. From 1996 to 1998, there was a 10 percent increase in illicit drug use among 12- to 17-year-olds. From 1999 to 2001, there was a 10.2 percent increase and from 2002 to 2004, an 8.6 percent decrease was noted.[22]

An interesting finding from the data in Table 2.3 is unrelated to the target but will be relevant in a later discussion. The percentage of young people reporting illicit drug use went up until 12th grade and then decreases among college students and young adults, such that the percentages are between those of 10th and 12th graders. This "maturing out" of drug use will be important as prevention efforts are discussed later in this book.

The finding that decreases in illicit drug use diminish and eventually reverse as survey participants get older suggests that the age of initiation of drug use may be increasing since 1996. In other words, 8th and 10th graders may be waiting until they are older to begin using drugs. This would explain the increases in percentages among older students and young adults. The issue of delaying the age of initiation of drug use is an important topic and will be discussed in this chapter.

Since the NDCS has emphasized the use of marijuana among young people, it is important to see if the changes in illicit drug use are related to the focus on marijuana. Tables 2.4 and 2.5 display these data from the Monitoring the Future Study. (The two final rows of these tables relate to the Bush goals in the 2002 NDCS and will be discussed later in this chapter).

For 8th and 10th graders, the decreases in any illicit drug use (Table 2.3) and any illicit drug use other than marijuana (Table 2.4) were quite similar. Therefore, for these two groups, the reductions in the rate of illicit drug use did not appear to be simply the result of decreased marijuana use. In fact, the decreases in marijuana use for 8th and 10th graders (Table 2.5) were very similar to the decreases in any illicit drugs other than marijuana, suggesting a consistency in reductions in 30-day use across different illicit drugs. However, the trend was different for 12th graders. This group showed substantial increases in illicit drug use other than marijuana from 1996 to 2002 and beyond. However, there was a much smaller increase in marijuana use from 1996 to 2002 and a decrease of over 9 percent from 1996 to 2005. For college students and young adults, there were substantial increases in illicit drug use other than marijuana over the 9-year period but much smaller increases in marijuana use. It would seem possible that the effect of delaying the initiation of illicit drug use other than marijuana rapidly deteriorates as students get older and is more than counteracted by substantial increases in adulthood. In fact, the rate of use of illicit drugs other than marijuana by college students and young adults in 1996 was lower than that of 8th graders. By 2004, the rate was higher than that of 10th graders. With regard to marijuana use, the effect of delaying the initiation of use deteriorated much more slowly. It may be that the impact of the NDCS activities has been more effective with regard to marijuana use than on the use of other illicit drugs. This issue is important as the relative danger of marijuana compared to other illicit drugs is examined in Chapter 4.

Table 2.4

**30-Day Prevalence of Any Illicit Drug Use Other Than Marijuana,
Monitoring the Future**

	8th Grade	10th Grade	12th Grade	8th–12th Grades	College Students	Young Adults
1996	6.9	8.9	9.5	8.4	4.5	4.7
1997	6.0	8.8	10.7	8.5	6.8	5.5
1998	5.5	8.6	10.7	8.3	6.1	5.5
1999	5.5	8.6	10.4	8.2	6.4	6.0
2000	5.6	8.5	10.4	8.2	6.9	6.4
2001	5.5	8.7	11.0	8.4	7.5	7.0
2002	4.7	8.1	11.3	8.0	7.8	7.7
2003	4.7	6.9	10.4	7.3	8.2	8.3
2004	4.1	6.9	10.8	7.3	9.1	8.5
2005	4.1	6.4	10.3	6.9	NA	NA
1996–2002	−31.9	−9.0	+18.9	−4.8	+73.3	+63.8
1996–end	−40.6	−28.1	+8.4	−17.9	+102.2	+80.9
2000–2002	−16.1	−4.7	+8.6	−2.4	+13.0	+10.9
2000–end	−26.8	−24.7	−1.0	−15.9	+31.9	+32.8

Note: "End" refers to 2005 for 8th, 10th, and 12th graders and 2004 for college students and young adults.
Source: Johnston et al. 2005.

Returning to the first part of Target 2, the 20 percent reduction in illicit drug use by young people by 2002 was achieved for 8th graders, regardless of whether overall illicit drug use, illicit drug use other than marijuana, or marijuana alone is examined. The 50 percent reduction by 2007 is certainly possible, given the trends. The goal for 2002 has not been achieved for 10th or 12th graders and is not likely to be achieved in 2007. However, reductions in use were noted for 10th graders. When 8th–12th grade results are averaged, the 2002 goal was not met for any illicit drug use, any illicit drug use other than marijuana, or for marijuana. The 2007 goal is unlikely to be met. There was no support for progress on this target by looking at the data from the National Household Survey.

Target 2 also references alcohol and tobacco use by young people. The relevant information related to this target is contained in Tables 2.6 and 2.7.

With regard to alcohol, the 2002 target goal was achieved for 8th graders but not for any other age group. The 2007 goal may be hard to achieve for 8th graders. For the compiled group, the 2002 goal was not met and the 2007 goal will probably not be met. Since relatively little attention is devoted to alcohol in the NDCS, this is not particularly surprising.

Table 2.5
30-Day Prevalence of Marijuana, Monitoring the Future

	8th Grade	10th Grade	12th Grade	8th–12th Grades	College Students	Young Adults
1996	11.3	20.4	21.9	17.9	17.5	15.1
1997	10.2	20.5	23.7	18.1	17.7	15.0
1998	9.7	18.7	22.8	17.1	18.6	14.9
1999	9.7	19.4	23.1	17.4	20.7	15.6
2000	9.1	19.7	21.6	16.8	20.0	16.1
2001	9.2	19.8	22.4	17.1	20.2	16.7
2002	8.3	17.8	21.5	15.9	19.7	16.9
2003	7.5	17.0	21.2	15.2	19.3	17.3
2004	6.4	15.9	19.9	14.1	18.9	16.5
2005	6.6	15.2	19.8	13.9	NA	NA
1996–2002	−26.5	−12.7	+6.8	−11.2	+12.6	+11.9
1996–end	−41.6	−25.4	−9.6	−22.3	+8.0	+9.3
2000–2002	0.0	−2.6	0	−5.4	−1.5	+5.0
2000–end	−27.4	−22.8	−8.3	−17.3	−5.5	+2.5

Note: "End" refers to 2005 for 8th, 10th, and 12th graders and 2004 for college students and young adults.
Source: Johnston et al. 2005.

The most apparent difference between the percentages of use of alcohol compared to illicit drugs is the much higher alcohol use. For secondary age students, the percentages were nearly or more than double. For college students and young adults, the percentage of individuals using alcohol was more than triple the percentage of those using illicit drugs. These results are not remarkable given the availability of alcohol and the fact that some college students and young adults can drink legally.

In the area of tobacco use (looking at cigarette smoking), the 2002 target for 8th and 10th graders was achieved and was very close for 12th graders (for some reason, the target for tobacco was set 5 percent higher than for alcohol and illicit drugs). The 2007 target has already been met for 8th graders and 10th graders. It is unlikely to be achieved for 12th graders. For the compiled group of 8th–12th graders, the 2002 goal was met and the 2007 goal is certainly possible.

Ironically, the data regarding youth use of tobacco is the most encouraging of any of the survey information; yet very few of the NDCS activities or initiatives involve tobacco. This is the only substance for which the target was achieved for the average of the 8th–12th graders and for which the 2007 target is within range.

Table 2.6
30-Day Prevalence of Any Alcohol Use, Monitoring the Future

	8th Grade	10th Grade	12th Grade	8th–12th Grades	College Students	Young Adults
1996	26.2	40.4	50.8	39.1	67.0	66.7
1997	24.5	40.1	52.7	39.1	65.8	67.5
1998	23.0	38.8	52.0	37.9	68.1	66.9
1999	24.0	40.0	51.0	38.3	69.6	68.2
2000	22.4	41.0	50.0	37.8	67.4	66.8
2001	21.5	39.0	49.8	36.8	67.0	67.0
2002	19.6	35.4	48.6	34.5	68.9	68.3
2003	19.7	35.4	47.5	34.2	66.2	67.0
2004	18.6	35.2	48.0	33.9	67.7	68.4
2005	17.1	33.2	47.0	32.4	NA	NA
1996–2002	−25.2	−12.4	−4.3	−11.8	+2.8	+2.4
1996–end	−34.7	−17.8	−7.5	−17.1	+1.0	+2.5

Note: "End" refers to 2005 for 8th, 10th, and 12th graders and 2004 for college students and young adults.
Source: Johnston et al. 2005.

Table 2.7
30-Day Prevalence of Cigarettes, Monitoring the Future

	8th Grade	10th Grade	12th Grade	8th–12th Grades	College Students	Young Adults
1996	21.0	30.4	34.0	28.5	27.9	30.1
1997	19.4	29.8	36.5	28.6	28.3	29.9
1998	19.1	27.6	35.1	27.3	30.0	30.9
1999	17.5	25.7	34.6	25.9	30.6	30.3
2000	14.6	23.9	31.4	23.3	28.2	30.1
2001	12.2	21.3	29.5	21.0	25.7	30.2
2002	10.7	17.7	26.7	18.4	26.7	29.2
2003	10.2	16.7	24.4	17.1	22.5	28.4
2004	9.2	16.0	25.0	16.7	24.3	29.2
2005	9.3	14.9	23.2	15.8	NA	NA
1996–2002	−49.0	−41.8	−21.5	−35.4	−4.3	−3.0
1996–end	−55.7	−51.0	−31.8	−44.6	−12.9	−3.0

Note: "End" refers to 2005 for 8th, 10th, and 12th graders and 2004 for college students and young adults.
Source: Johnston et al. 2005.

I cannot explain why a reduction in tobacco use among youth was included in the targets in the 1999 NDCS.

It is also interesting that tobacco use among college students and young adults has decreased over the survey period, in contrast to the data on illicit drugs. The most likely explanation involves the changes in tobacco policies that have taken place since 1996. This will be explored in detail in Chapter 6 where substance abuse prevention is discussed.

Before moving on to Target 3, there is a question that must be addressed: What is so important about reducing 30-day prevalence of illicit drug use? It is important to answer this question because 30-day prevalence is not just the focus of Targets 1 and 2 but it is the *only* goal in the Bush administration's NDCS.

The answer to this question may seem obvious to you. Kids who are using drugs, even occasionally, may develop drug addiction or suffer consequences related to drug use. For example, the 2002 NDCS cited information from the 2002 National Household Survey that adults 18 or older who tried marijuana at age 14 or younger were nearly five times more likely to be classified as drug dependent or have a drug abuse problem than adults who first used marijuana at age 18 or older.[23]

Here is the issue. In statistics, there is an old cliché "Correlation does not imply causation." This means that just because two events occur together, it doesn't mean that one causes the other. For example, if I tell you that convicted felons consume more mashed potatoes than non felons, it doesn't mean that eating mashed potatoes causes crime. There is probably an intervening factor that explains the relationship (i.e., mashed potatoes are served frequently in prison).

So, it is not clear if starting to use marijuana at age 14 or earlier causes addiction or if there is another explanation for the relationship. Perhaps young people who start using marijuana at an early age have a greater likelihood of a family history of addiction. There is a well-established genetic component to addiction. Furthermore, if family members are actively using alcohol and other drugs, these children would have more exposure and access to drugs than other children. Perhaps young people who start smoking marijuana in early adolescence have a number of risk factors for substance abuse (e.g., peers who use, deprivation, school failure, neglect and abuse), the combination of which increases the probability of later dependence or abuse.

What the 2002 NDCS strategy does not mention is that the National Household Survey found that only 13 percent of children who started to use marijuana at age 14 or earlier developed a substance dependence or abuse problem. So, 87 percent didn't. Looking at the differences between those who developed substance abuse problems later in life and those who did not would probably tell us something about whether delaying the age of initiation of drug use has any value in preventing the incidence of later dependence or abuse.

A personal example may illustrate this point. I still maintain contact with seven childhood friends. We started playing poker in 9th grade and we continue to have an annual game. I have known most of these guys since elementary school and all of them since 7th grade. We graduated from high school in 1969, so there were a lot of drugs around, especially marijuana and hallucinogens. We did our share of experimenting. We also did a lot of drinking. Some of us are professionals today, others are blue collar. Some did really well in school; others were mediocre students. No one got into any serious trouble but we weren't model citizens. Today, I am the only one with an alcohol or drug problem. The other guys drink moderately and none of them use any illicit drugs. I am also the only one with a family history of alcoholism.

Although one case like this doesn't prove anything, it does illustrate the point. Most young people who use drugs do not develop later problems. As the Monitoring the Future Survey results showed, prevalence falls after high school. There is a "maturing out" of drug use. Perhaps the 8th and 10th graders who delayed their use until later were like the rest of my poker friends. Even if they had started using drugs at an earlier age, they would not have experienced problems later anyway. They would have "matured out" of their drug use as they got older.

Exploring some other data can help determine if this possibility has any support. For example, the Monitoring the Future Survey does ask about daily use of marijuana. (The survey also gathers information on the daily use of alcohol and tobacco. The daily use of other drugs by students is too small to be measured with any meaning.)

Now, young people who are smoking marijuana every day have a substance abuse problem in my opinion. I would say the same thing about someone who is drinking to the point of euphoria every day. It is reasonable to expect that if delaying the age of initiation of marijuana use has an impact on the development of later marijuana abuse or dependence, there should be a decreasing number of daily marijuana users, especially among college students and young adults.

As can be seen from Table 2.8, the opposite is true. The prevalence of daily use has increased from 12th grade on. It is hard to make much of the changes in 8th grade since the prevalence is so low. For 10th graders, there really has not been any significant change since 1996, with the prevalence remarkably stable except in 2001. When the average is calculated for 8th–12th graders, there was more than a 12 percent increase in daily marijuana use from 1996 to 2002 and some decrease from 1996 to 2005.

Some would argue that detecting the impact of delaying the age of initiation of marijuana requires looking at substance abuse or dependence rates over many years since these problems may not be evidenced until later adulthood. Unfortunately, there is no way to look at these data for the 1996 8th and 10th graders since

Table 2.8
Daily Use of Marijuana, Monitoring the Future

	8th Grade	10th Grade	12th Grade	8th–12th Grades	College Students	Young Adults
1996	1.5	3.5	4.9	3.3	2.8	3.3
1997	1.1	3.7	5.8	3.5	3.7	3.8
1998	1.1	3.6	5.6	3.4	4.0	3.7
1999	1.4	3.8	6.0	3.7	4.0	4.4
2000	1.3	3.8	6.0	3.7	4.6	4.2
2001	1.3	4.5	5.8	3.9	4.5	5.0
2002	1.2	3.9	6.0	3.7	4.1	4.5
2003	1.0	3.6	6.0	3.5	4.7	5.3
2004	0.8	3.2	5.6	3.2	4.5	5.0
2005	1.0	3.1	5.0	3.0	NA	NA
1996–2002	−20.0	+11.4	+22.4	+12.1	+46.4	+36.4
1996–end	−33.3	−11.4	+2.0	−9.1	+60.7	+51.5

Note: "End" refers to 2005 for 8th, 10th, and 12th graders and 2004 for college students and young adults.
Source: Johnston et al. 2005.

they would be only 21 to 24 years old by 2004. Only the available data can be examined to determine if there is any support for the hypothesis that delaying the age of initiation of marijuana use would result in lower rates of marijuana abuse of dependence in adulthood. Thus far, this hypothesis does not have data to support it.

However, delaying the age of initiation of drug use may also reduce the unintended harm that can result from drug use, such as overdoses, accidents, and risky behavior. There is some data on these areas that will be discussed under Target 12.

Target 3. Increase the average age of first-time drug use by twelve months by 2002 and thirty-six months by 2007.

It should be noted that the data from 1996 to 2002 were derived from the 2002 and 2003 National Household Survey by asking participants when they first used these substances. Therefore, it is acceptable to compare across these years. In the 2004 survey, the procedures to determine age of first use were changed so the 2003 and 2004 data must be compared to earlier years with caution.

As can be seen from Table 2.9, this goal had not been achieved by 2002. The average age of first use of marijuana was virtually the same as in 1996 while the average age of first use of cocaine, hallucinogens, and ecstasy had gone down.

Table 2.9
Average Age of First Use of Drugs: National Household Survey

	Marijuana	Cocaine	Hallucinogens	Ecstasy	Pain Medication
1996	16.9	21.9	19.1	21.9	21.4
1997	17.2	20.8	19.0	20.8	22.0
1998	17.0	20.8	19.0	20.8	23.2
1999	17.5	20.8	18.7	20.8	22.4
2000	16.9	20.9	18.7	20.9	22.1
2001	17.3	20.8	19.3	20.8	21.0
2002	17.2	20.3	18.3	20.3	22.2
2003	17.5	19.8	17.9	19.7	24.0
2004	18.0	20.0	18.7	19.5	23.3

Sources: Office of Applied Studies, Substance Abuse and Mental Health Services Administration. 2004. National Survey on Drug Use and Health. Appendix G: Selected prevalence tables. http://oas.samhsa.gov/NHSDA/2k3NSDUH/appg.htm#tabg.35; Office of Applied Studies, Substance Abuse and Mental Health Services Administration. 2005. National Survey on Drug Use and Health. Appendix H: Selected prevalence tables. http://oas.samhsa.gov/nsduh/2k4nsduh/2k4Results/appH.htm#tabh.32.

The average age of first, nonmedical use of prescription pain medications has increased nearly 1 year but there were no consistent trends in these data. Even with the cautions about comparing the 2003 and 2004 data with earlier years, there is virtually no chance that the 2007 goals will be met.

Since marijuana is the primary illicit substance used by all age groups and it is assumed that this target is primarily concerned with increasing the first time age of marijuana use, data from another survey will be examined; the Youth Risk Behavior Surveillance Survey (YRBSS). This survey of 9th through 12th graders is conducted by the Centers for Disease Control on a biannual basis to determine the prevalence of high-risk behaviors among youth.[24] One question on the survey involves the percentage of students who tried marijuana for the first time before age 13. The results from the YRBSS were as follows[25]:

1997	9.7%
1999	11.3%
2001	10.2%
2003	9.9%
2005	8.7%

From 1997 to 2005, there has been a 10 percent decrease in the number of students under 13 who had tried marijuana for the first time. While the trend is in a favorable direction and consistent with the data in Table 2.9, it would not appear to be large enough to provide evidence that Target 3 will be achieved by 2007. Clearly, the 2002 target was not met.

Finally, in the 2004 National Household Survey, the average age of first use of marijuana for all first-time users who began to use marijuana before the age of 21 was computed. The average age in 2002 was 15.9, 15.9 in 2003, and 16.0 in 2004.[26] Therefore, the increase in the average age of first use of marijuana from 2002 to 2004 seen in Table 2.9 would appear to be to due to delays in the age of initiation of marijuana by some people to age 21 and older. This would be consistent with the trends noted earlier in the increasing age of initiation of illicit drug use among some young people.

Target 4. Reduce the prevalence of drug use in the workplace by 25 percent by 2002 and 50 percent by 2007.

In the 1999 NDCS, there is a reference to the number of employed drug users and a table of data from the National Household Survey regarding the employment status of illicit drug users. Unfortunately, as was seen before in looking at this survey, comparisons across years are not possible because of the changes in the survey procedures. However, these data can be examined to determine if there is any evidence to support this target.

There is no evidence to support progress on Target 4. If you will recall, survey results from 1996 to 1998, from 1999 to 2001, and from 2002 to 2003 can be compared. For full-time employees, the only decrease in use that can be found was from 2002 to 2003 in any illicit drug use. This decrease was 3.6 percent. For part-time employees, there was a considerable decrease in any illicit drug use from 1996 to 1998 but a greater increase from 1999 to 2001. A decrease in cocaine use from 1996 to 1998 was followed by an increase from 1999 to 2001.

Target 5. Reduce the number of chronic drug users by 20 percent by 2002 and 50 percent by 2007.

In the 1999 NDCS, the narrative of this target mentions an "... estimated 3.6 million chronic cocaine users and 810,000 chronic heroin users."[27] However, there is no reference for these data. The National Household Survey began asking questions in 2000 reflecting past year substance abuse or dependence. From 2000 to 2001, the percentage of people reporting past year substance abuse or dependence increased from 1.9 percent to 2.5 percent.[28] From 2002 to 2004, the percentages remained stable (3.0 in 2002 and 3.0 in 2004).[29] Although there is no accurate baseline from 1996, there also is no evidence of progress on this target.

Table 2.10
Drug Use by Employment Status: National Household Surveys

	Full-Time	Part-Time	Unemployed	Other
Past month: any illicit drug				
1996	6.2	8.6	12.5	3.0
1997	6.5	7.7	13.8	3.0
1998	6.4	7.4	18.2	2.8
1999	6.1	8.2	16.2	3.3
2000	6.3	7.7	16.9	3.6
2001	6.9	9.1	17.1	3.9
2002	8.2	10.5	17.4	4.9
2003	7.9	10.7	18.2	4.8
Past month: marijuana				
1996	4.9	6.2	10.0	2.3
1997	5.0	6.6	12.2	2.4
1998	5.1	6.5	15.1	2.0
1999	4.7	6.6	12.1	2.2
2000	4.8	6.2	14.4	2.6
2001	5.4	7.6	14.1	2.5
2002	6.2	8.3	12.7	3.6
2003	6.3	8.4	13.8	3.0
Past month: cocaine				
1996	0.9	1.1	2.4	0.4
1997	0.7	0.9	2.4	0.3
1998	0.9	0.5	3.4	0.4
1999	0.8	0.8	2.9	0.3
2000	0.5	0.9	1.8	0.3
2001	0.8	1.1	3.5	0.4
2002	0.8	1.1	2.7	0.7
2003	1.1	1.3	2.7	0.4

Note: All data except 2003 taken from compilation included in the 2004 NDCS. 2003 data are from the National Household Survey.
Sources: Office of National Drug Control Policy. 2004. The President's national drug control strategy: Data supplement. http://www.whitehousedrugpolicy.gov/publications/policy/ndcs04/data_suppl.htm.; Office of Applied Studies 2005.

Substance use goals established by the Bush administration: The 2-year goals (2000–2002) in the first NDCS issued by the Bush administration in 2002 were to reduce illegal drug use by 12- to 17-year-olds and by adults by 10 percent. The 5-year goals were for 25 percent reductions in these same groups. Illegal drug use was defined as any use of illicit drugs in the past month. The time period of the goal was somewhat odd since the first Bush NDCS was issued in 2002. So any changes from 2000 to 2002 would reflect the Clinton NDCS.

Although data from the National Household Survey are not totally useful because of the changes in survey procedures, these data do not support the goal, as can be seen from Table 2.2. In the 12- to 17-year-age group, use of any illicit drug went up from 2000 to 2001 and went down 8.6 from 2002 to 2004. In the 12 and older group, the same trend was noted, with a smaller decrease of 4.8 percent from 2002 to 2004.

The data from the Monitoring the Future study (Tables 2.3–2.5) do provide some evidence to support the 2-year and 5-year goals for 12- to 17-year-olds, although not for young adults. For 8th graders, the 2-year and 5-year goals have been achieved for any illicit drug and any illicit drug other than marijuana. The 2-year goal for marijuana was nearly achieved for the 8th graders and the 5-year goal has already been achieved. For 10th graders, the trends were definitely in the expected direction for both 2-year and 5-year goals. The 12th graders had not achieved any of the goals. In fact, their use of illicit drugs except marijuana is virtually unchanged from 2000 to 2005. The combined average for 8th–12th graders showed that the 2-year goal was not met. The 5-year goals are possible but not likely.

College students and young adults did not achieve any of the goals and showed large increases in their use of illicit drugs other than marijuana.

In summary, the two goals of the 2002 NDCS were not achieved for 12- to 17-year-olds as a group or for young adults. If 12- to 17-year-olds are looked at by age groups, there was certainly more progress for younger adolescents. The 5-year goals will probably not be met for 12- to 17-year-olds, although there has been a reduction in 30-day use of illicit drugs. The 5-year goal will not be met for young adults.

Substance use targets established in the ONDCP Reauthorization Act of 1998[30] :

1. Reduction of unlawful drug use to 3 percent or less of the U.S. population by December 31, 2003 (as measured in terms of overall illicit drug use during the past thirty days by National Household Survey on Drug Abuse (NHSDA)) and achievement of at least 20 percent of such reduction during 1999, 2000, 2001, 2002, and 2003, respectively.

This target has not been achieved. In Table 2.2, 7.9 percent of the U.S. population reported using illicit drugs in the past month, according to the 2004 National Household Survey. Even with the changes in survey procedures, there have not been any years approaching the 20 percent progress toward the goal. From 1999 to 2000, there was no change. From 2000 to 2001, there was a 12.7 percent increase. The results from 2001 to 2002 cannot be compared because of the survey procedure changes. From 2002 to 2004, there was a 4.8 percent decrease.

2. Reduction of unlawful adolescent drug use (as measured in terms of illicit drug use during the past thirty days by the Monitoring the Future (MTF) study of the University of Michigan or the National PRIDE survey conducted by the Parents' Resource Institute for Drug Education) to 3 percent or less of the U.S. adolescent population by December 31, 2003, and achievement of at least 20 percent of such reduction during 1999, 2000, 2001, 2002, and 2003, respectively.

This target was not achieved. In Table 2.3 (MTF survey), it can be seen that, in 2003, even 8th graders used illicit drugs at more than triple the rate of this goal. There was no year from 1999 on in which any age group showed the required 20 percent progress toward the goal.

On the PRIDE survey, monthly use of any illicit drugs was 15.1 percent in the 2002–2003 school year and 13.8 percent in the 2003–2004 school year, far higher than the target. [31]

Drug Availability Targets and Goals

Drug availability targets from the Clinton administration 1999 NDCS: The supply reduction targets will be discussed together since the relevant data sets relate to multiple targets.

Target 6. Reduce the domestic availability of illegal drugs by 25 percent in 2002 and 50 percent by 2007.

Target 7. Reduce the rate of shipment of illegal drugs from source countries by 15 percent by 2002 and 30 percent by 2007.

Target 8. Reduce the rate at which illegal drugs enter the United States by 10 percent by 2002 and 20 percent by 2007.

Target 9. Reduce the production of methamphetamine and cultivation of marijuana in the United States by 20 percent by 2002 and 50 percent by 2007.

Target 10. Reduce trafficker success rate in the United States. (In the target narrative, goals of a 10 percent reduction by 2002 and a 20 percent reduction by 2007 are mentioned).

According to the narrative in the 1999 NDCS report, there were no baseline measures for any drug except cocaine for Target 8, and no baseline measures for Targets 9 and 10. There were only indirect measures of Target 6. Obviously, this complicates the task of determining if progress toward these targets has occurred.

Table 2.11

Price of Illicit Drugs, Average Price Per Gram (Constant 2002 dollars)

	Cocaine	Crack	Heroin	Methamphetamine	Marijuana
1996	179.83	153.33	515.03	238.95	10.08
1997	154.28	165.55	493.94	195.42	9.34
1998	114.57	169.82	472.51	209.90	8.76
1999	145.02	256.25	415.09	254.13	9.79
2000	160.42	214.16	428.43	148.31	8.85
2001	166.44	227.09	391.98	175.86	9.67
2002	134.08	191.45	392.39	180.01	11.19
2003 (Q2)	94.12	159.63	362.14	167.79	11.33

Note: Data available through the second quarter of 2003.
Source: Office of National Drug Control Policy 2004. The price and purity of illicit drugs: 1981 through the second quarter of 2003.

One way to indirectly assess progress toward supply reduction targets is to examine the price and purity of illicit drugs. If the availability of illicit drugs is reduced by eradication, seizures, and arrests, an increase in the price and/or a decrease in the purity of illicit drugs would be expected. However, as noted in the 1999 NDCS report

> Variations in wholesale and retail prices and purities of drugs are indirect and often inaccurate estimates of availability as a result of their dependence on both supply and demand. Reduced supply, for example, would result in higher prices and lower purity levels were demand to remain constant. Conversely, reduced demand and constant supply would result in lower prices and higher purity levels.[32]

As has been seen, demand has not decreased. Therefore, price and purity should be good indicators of availability of illicit drugs. This information is shown in Tables 2.11 and 2.12.

The price of cocaine is nearly 48 percent less in 2003 than it was in 1996, with the purity virtually unchanged. Neither the price nor purity of crack has changed over this time, although there was a price spike from 1999 to 2002. The price of heroin has decreased nearly 30 percent. Except for the drop in purity in the second quarter of 2003, purity has been fairly stable. The price of methamphetamine has decreased nearly 30 percent and the purity has increased by nearly a quarter. The price of marijuana has increased over 12 percent. However, the THC content

Table 2.12
Purity Per Gram of Illicit Drugs and Potency of Marijuana

	Cocaine	Crack	Heroin	Methamphetamine	Marijuana
1996	0.68	0.78	0.37	0.52	4.50
1997	0.69	0.78	0.45	0.67	5.00
1998	0.75	0.76	0.44	0.54	4.89
1999	0.62	0.70	0.41	0.36	4.59
2000	0.63	0.69	0.44	0.46	5.34
2001	0.60	0.69	0.39	0.52	6.11
2002	0.65	0.70	0.46	0.64	7.19
2003 (Q2)	0.69	0.75	0.29	0.64	7.12

Notes: Except for marijuana, data available through the second quarter of 2003. Marijuana data was available through 2003. The data for marijuana refers to the THC potency.
Sources: Office of National Drug Control Policy 2004. The price and purity of illicit drugs: 1981 through the second quarter of 2003; Office of National Drug Control Policy 2004. The President's national drug control strategy: Data supplement.

of marijuana (the active ingredient of marijuana that determines potency) has increased by over 58 percent.

With the exception of a decrease in the purity of heroin in the second quarter of 2003 and an increase in the price of high potency marijuana, these data do not support any of the supply reduction targets. Certainly, these data suggest that the availability of illicit drugs is at least stable and perhaps increasing (Target 6). It is highly unlikely that these price and purity data would exist if the shipment of illegal drugs from source countries was decreasing (Target 7), if the rate at which illegal drugs were entering the country was decreasing (Target 8), if the production of methamphetamine and cultivation of marijuana was reduced (Target 9), or if traffickers were having less and less success (Target 10).

There is another comprehensive, federal data source on these targets. Since 2001, the National Drug Intelligence Center in the U.S. Department of Justice has published a report titled, "National Drug Threat Assessment."[33] The availability of each type of illicit drug is discussed. The following information is from the various reports:

Cocaine

2001: "Law enforcement agencies throughout the nation generally agree that cocaine availability remains high . . . Cocaine and crack continue to consume the resources of law enforcement and the justice system . . . Federal-wide

Drug Seizure System (FDSS) data show a significant increase in cocaine seizures from 1998 to 1999 ... Law enforcement agencies in urban areas report that crack remains readily available."[34]

2002: "High demand for and availability of the drug, expansion of cocaine distribution markets, high rates of overdose and collateral crimes, and endemic violence all contribute to the magnitude of the threat. Countering the threat posed by cocaine consumes enormous domestic counterdrug resources, particularly since international cocaine trafficking organizations have demonstrated an ability to modify trafficking operations, shift smuggling routes, and improve concealment techniques in response to multinational interdiction efforts."[35]

2003: "Both powder cocaine and crack are prevalent throughout the country, and overall availability is stable at high levels ... Statistical reporting regarding cocaine-related federal investigations, arrests, and seizures did not change appreciably from 2000 to 2001 ... Estimated cocaine production increased in 2001, however, estimates suggest that only about 28 percent of the export-quality cocaine prepared for shipment to world markets was smuggled into the United States ..."[36]

2004: "Worldwide cocaine production decreased significantly in 2002, largely because of intensified coca eradication in Colombia ... The distribution of powder cocaine and crack cocaine occurs throughout the country, and the market for the drug appears to be stable overall."[37]

2005: "Key indicators show stable or slightly increased cocaine availability in the U.S. drug markets despite sharp decreases in the amount of cocaine transported toward the United States from South America in 2003 ... Worldwide cocaine production has decreased sharply since 2001, primarily because of a 34 percent decline in cocaine production in Colombia from 700 metric tons in 2001 to 460 metric tons in 2003."[38]

Methamphetamine

2001: "Law enforcement agencies generally agree that availability is high ... Federal-wide Drug Seizure System data show that over 2,700 kilograms of methamphetamine were seized in 1999—approximately 200 kilograms more than were seized in 1998."[39]

2002: "Methamphetamine is readily available throughout the western half of the country and is becoming increasingly available in areas of the eastern United States."[40]

2003: "Reporting from law enforcement and public health agencies indicates that methamphetamine availability is widespread in the western and central United States and is increasing in the eastern half of the country, albeit slowly. Despite overall increasing availability and an increase in methamphetamine seized, data regarding methamphetamine-related federal investigations and arrests show decreases in 2001. These decreases likely are due to a shift by DEA to investigate fewer but higher priority methamphetamine targets."[41]

2004: "Methamphetamine availability is very high in the Pacific, South-west, and West Central regions. In the Great Lakes and Southeast regions, methamphetamine availability has increased to such a level that most state and local law enforcement agencies now report that availability of the drug is either high or moderate in their areas. Methamphetamine availability in the Northeast/Mid-Atlantic region is low but increasing. Despite wide-ranging reports of increasing availability, the number of methamphetamine-related Organized Crime Drug Enforcement Task Force investigations and Drug Enforcement Administration arrests, as well as the amount of methamphetamine seized by federal agencies, all decreased from 2001 to 2002 . . . Domestic methamphetamine production appears to be increasing . . . the Drug Enforcement Administration reports that methamphetamine production in Mexico—the primary foreign source area for the drug—appears to have increased. "[42]

2005: "Methamphetamine availability has increased sharply over the past year in the Northeast Region, primarily because of an increase in whole-sale distribution by Mexican criminal groups . . . National-level laboratory seizure data as well as law enforcement reporting indicated that domestic methamphetamine production has expanded to more areas of the country . . . Law enforcement reporting and drug seizure data indicated that methamphetamine production has increased sharply in Mexico since 2002."[43]

Heroin

2001: "According to the FDSS, federal seizures declined from almost 1,500 kilograms in 1998 to just over 1,100 kilograms in 1999 . . . Law enforcement agencies throughout the country note that heroin is readily available . . . Heroin purity has increased dramatically in the past 10 years while prices have fallen—both primary indicators of increased availability."[44]

2002: "The drug is widely available, and the user population is growing to include an increasing number of young people . . . Heroin from all major sources—South America, Mexico, Southeast Asia, and Southwest Asia—is available in various locations throughout the country."[45]

2003: "Reporting from law enforcement and public health agencies indicates that the availability of heroin is widespread and that it is increasing, particularly in New England in areas of the Mid-Atlantic."[46]

2004: "Law enforcement reporting indicates that heroin remains readily available throughout most major metropolitan areas, and availability is increasing in many suburban and rural areas . . . Estimates of worldwide heroin production increased considerably between 2001 and 2002 primarily because of increases in Afghanistan—a primary source of heroin destined for Europe. Heroin production estimates for Colombia and Mexico decreased, however."[47]

2005: "The availability of Southwest Asian heroin appears to have increased slightly in 2003; however, preliminary 2004 data indicate that availability of Southwest Asian heroin may be declining to pre-2003 levels. Worldwide heroin production increased in 2002, 2003, and 2004, attributable overwhelmingly to increases in production in Afghanistan."[48]

Marijuana

2001: " The availability of high-grade marijuana is increasing in every region, and some regions report the price is decreasing . . . Despite beliefs that the threat of marijuana is overshadowed by concern with other illegal drugs, federal data show that efforts to stem the trafficking of marijuana continue to consume the resources of federal, state, and local agencies and the judicial system. Marijuana seizures reflected in the FDSS rose from almost 828,000 kilograms in 1998 to approximately 1.1 million kilograms in 1999. "[49]

2002: "The ready availability and popularity of marijuana render the drug a significant threat to the country . . . The demand for marijuana far exceeds that for any other illicit drug, and the large user populations in the United States equates to steady profits for traffickers. The profit potential is so high that drug trafficking organizations, criminal groups, and gangs involved in trafficking drugs such as cocaine and heroin traffic marijuana as well to help finance their drug operations."[50]

2003: "It is the most readily available and widely used illicit drug in the United States . . . Available data suggest that marijuana production is high both in the United States and in foreign source areas . . . Distribution of marijuana appears to be stable . . ."[51]

2004: "The availability of marijuana is stable at high levels ... Drug markets across the country are supplied with significant quantities of marijuana produced in foreign source areas (chiefly Mexico, but also Canada, Colombia, and Jamaica) as well as domestically. Marijuana transportation and subsequent distribution by a wide range of criminal groups, gangs, and independent dealers are commonplace throughout the country, resulting in an overall domestic market for marijuana that is strong and stable."[52]

2005: "Domestic marijuana production appears to be increasing, in part because of the rising involvement of U.S.-based Mexican criminal groups in domestic cultivation. Mexico has been the principal source area for U.S.-destined foreign marijuana for decades, and already high production levels escalated in 2003. An estimated 13,500 metric tons of marijuana were potentially produced in Mexico in 2003—70 percent more than in the previous year."[53]

When the data from Tables 2.11 and 2.12 are combined with the narrative reports from the National Drug Threat Assessments, it is very clear that Target 6 has not been achieved. In fact, no progress has been made on reducing the domestic availability of illegal drugs. There has been a reduction in the production of cocaine in Colombia, which presumably would lead to a conclusion that there has been progress on reducing the shipment of illegal drugs (at least with regard to cocaine) from source countries (Target 7). However, the National Drug Threat Assessments indicate that production of heroin, methamphetamine, and marijuana in source countries has been stable or has increased. Since the National Drug Threat Assessment noted that cocaine has remained readily available in spite of the production reductions in Colombia, it is logical to conclude that the rate at which this drug has entered the United States has not been reduced (Target 8) or that there has been a reduction in trafficker success (Target 10). With regard to methamphetamine, heroin, and marijuana, the National Drug Threat Assessment reports indicated that there has been no progress on Targets 8 and 10. Finally, the National Drug Threat Assessments found that production of methamphetamine and cultivation of marijuana has been increasing. Therefore, no progress has been made on Target 9.

Drug availability targets established in the ONDCP Reauthorization Act of 1998:

3. Reduction of cocaine, heroin, marijuana, and methamphetamine availability in the United States by 80 percent by December 31, 2003.

This target has not been achieved. According to the National Drug Threat Assessment reports, the availability of all of these illicit substances has remained high.

4. Reduction of nationwide average street purity levels for cocaine, heroin, marijuana, and methamphetamine (as estimated by the interagency drug-flow assessment process, the Drug Enforcement Administration, and other national drug-control program agencies) by 60 percent by December 31, 2003, and achievement of at least 20 percent of such reduction during 1999, 2000, 2001, 2002, and 2003, respectively.

This target has not been achieved. From Table 2.12, it can be seen that the only illicit substance with a significant decrease in purity was heroin and that decrease occurred from 2002 to the second quarter of 2003. The purity of methamphetamine and the potency of marijuana have increased.

Targets and Goals Related to the Consequences of Drug Abuse

Targets related to the consequences of drug abuse from the Clinton administration 1999 NDCS:

Target 11. Reduce crime associated with drug trafficking and use by 15 percent by 2002 and 30 percent by 2007.

There is no direct data source to determine crime associated with drug use. The 1999 NDCS report does make reference to the number of arrests for drug law violations in 1996 and a determination can be made if this has changed over time.

While the percentage of all arrests that involve drug abuse violations has increased from 1996 to 2002, the absolute number of drug abuse arrests has also increased by a little more than 2 percent. It is also clear that increases in drug abuse arrests do not involve an enhanced effort to apprehend drug traffickers rather than drug users. The percentage of all drug abuse violations that involve drug possession was actually lower in 1996 than in any subsequent year.

Crime has definitely decreased in the United States from 1996 to 2002.[54] This includes violent crimes and property crimes. However, the relationship between this decrease and drug abuse is unknown. There has been a decrease of about 12 percent in total number of crime incidents from 1996 to 2002. At the same time, there has been an increase of more than 20 percent in the number of people who were in prison during this same time period.[55] Therefore, it is reasonable to suspect that the increased number of incarcerated individuals has contributed to a reduction in crimes.

Table 2.13
Drug Arrests from 1996 to 2002

	% of Arrests for Drug Abuse Violations	% of Drug Abuse Arrests for Possession
1996	9.9	75.2
1997	10.3	79.5
1998	10.7	78.8
1999	10.9	80.4
2000	10.9	78.7
2001	11.5	80.6
2002	11.2	77.2

Note: 2002 was the last year data available at the time this was prepared.
Source: Office of National Drug Control Policy. 2004. The President's national drug control strategy: Data supplement. 48.

An indirect measure of Target 11 involves the crime-related costs of drug abuse. In Chapter 1, reference was made to a study of the economic costs of drug abuse, commissioned by ONDCP. In 1996 the crime-related costs of drug abuse were estimated to be $78.4 billion. In 2002, these costs were estimated to be $107.8 billion.[56]

Finally, the National Institute of Justice had a program called the Arrestee Drug Abuse Monitoring (ADAM) program. ADAM involved conducting urinalysis of arrestees at 35 sites across the country. There are annual reports covering the arrestees from 1997 to 2003 but they are not uniform in format and content. The 1997 report stated that, "Every site reported that a majority of its male adult arrestees tested positive for at least one drug."[57] In the report of the 2003 cohort, 67 percent of male arrestees tested positive. Only one site (Woodbury, Iowa) had less than 50 percent of male arrestees test positive and only two other sites had less than 60 percent.[58] While it is very risky to draw any firm conclusions from this information, it would not be consistent with a reduction in drug-related crime during this time period.

Target 12. Reduce the health and social costs associated with drug trafficking and use by 10 percent by 2002 and 25 percent by 2007.

The only data mentioned in the narrative of the 1999 NDCS for this target involves cases of tuberculosis that were drug related. However, there are some data sources available that provide direct and indirect measures of this target.

The health and social costs in economic terms have been calculated by ONDCP in a study that has been referenced previously, "The Economic Costs of Drug Abuse in the United States: 1992–2002."[59] The overall costs of drug abuse in 1996 were estimated to be $129.6 billion and $180.8 billion in 2002, an increase of nearly 40 percent. In the study, these figures were also calculated in terms of constant 2002 dollars to account for inflation. In this case, the increase was a little over 20 percent.

The 2004 NDCS report also has some data related to this target. The number of deaths from drug-induced causes rose from 14,843 in 1996 to 21,683 in 2002, an increase of over 46 percent.[60] The death rate per 100,000 population from drug-induced causes rose from 5.6 in 1996 to 7.6 in 2001 (last year reported), an increase of nearly 36 percent.[61] The number of injecting drug users living with AIDS has increased by over 45 percent between 1996 and 2002.[62] From 1996 to 2002, the total number of drug episodes in emergency rooms increased over 30 percent and total drug mentions in emergency rooms increased over 33 percent. Of the drugs mentioned in emergency rooms, cocaine increased nearly 31 percent, heroin increased over 28 percent, and marijuana mentions increased more than 122 percent.[63]

Since tuberculosis was mentioned in the narrative of the 1999 NDCS report regarding this target, these data should be examined. The percentage of injecting drug users of the total number of tuberculosis cases has dropped from 3.8 percent to 2.2 percent from 1996 to 2002, a drop of over 42 percent. The percentage of total tuberculosis cases of noninjecting drug users has dropped from 7.7 percent to 7.0 percent, a drop of 10 percent.[64] It may be that needle exchange programs, in which injecting drug users can exchange used syringes for new ones, in urban areas have contributed to this improvement among injecting drug users because tuberculosis screening is frequently offered as a part of needle exchange programs. However, ONDCP is opposed to needle exchange programs and these programs exist without any federal support.

For adolescents and young adults, most of the data on social and health costs are indirect since the frequency of occurrence of death, AIDS, and other direct consequences are so low among young people. However, emergency room mentions from adolescents and young adults through data collected by the Drug Abuse Warning Network (DAWN), a federally sponsored system involving 21 metropolitan areas, can be looked at. This is the same source for the emergency room data discussed earlier. (In 2003, the DAWN data collection system was changed. Therefore, data from 2003 on cannot be compared to earlier data).

The data in this table reflect the frequency at which drugs were mentioned during emergency room visits. It does not imply that only that particular drug

Table 2.14
Emergency Room Mentions per 100,000 Population, 1996 to 2002

	12- to 17-year-olds		18- to 25-year-olds	
	1996	**2002**	**1996**	**2002**
Alcohol in combination with drugs	29	32	100	113
Marijuana	45	77	57	109
Cocaine	12	14	80	91
Heroin	2	3	33	52
Methamphetamine	5	5	14	17

Source: Substance Abuse and Mental Health Services Administration. 2003. Drug Abuse Warning Network (DAWN). http://dawninfo.samhsa.gov/old_dawn/pubs_94_02/pickatable/getpage.asp.

was mentioned or that the drug mentioned caused the emergency room visit. It can be seen that the prevalence of emergency room mentions has increased for all these categories and in both age groups, except for methamphetamine among 12- to 17-year-olds, which remained the same. The increases in marijuana mentions are quite large.

It should be noted that drug-related emergency room episodes (actual number of drug-related emergency room visits, regardless of the number of drugs mentioned) decreased by 10.2 percent for 12- to 17-year-olds during this time period and increased by 15.6 percent in the 18–25 age category.

The indirect data on the social costs of drug abuse among youth is available from the YRBSS.[65] Again, because this survey is conducted biannually, 1997 will be used as the base year and 2005 as the end point.

Drank alcohol or used drugs before last sexual intercourse: down 5.7 percent

Sex with one or more people during past 3 months: down 2.6 percent

Sex for the first time before age 13: down 13.9 percent

Injured in a physical fight: up 2.9 percent

In a physical fight: down 1.9 percent

Carried a gun in last month: down 8.5 percent

Carried any weapon in last month: up 1.1 percent

Threatened or injured with a weapon on school property: up 6.8 percent

Did not go to school in past month because felt unsafe: up 50.0 percent

Attempted suicide in past year: up 9.1 percent

Made a suicide plan in past year: down 17.2 percent

The YRBSS has much more information than what is reported here. These questions would be the most likely to be directly or indirectly related to drug use. Although some of these issues have moved in a positive direction, others have not. Sexual behaviors reduced somewhat and violence-related behaviors generally increased. Achievement of the 2007 goal is possible only in regard to suicide planning. However, suicide attempts have increased in the time frame reported.

Finally, school drop-out rate may have an indirect relationship to youth drug use since young people who abuse drugs are more likely to drop out of school than those who do not.[66] In the 2004 NDCS report, there is a table of annual drop-out rates compiled by the U.S. Bureau of the Census.[67] However, these data seem a bit odd. The drop-out rate in 1996 is reported to be 4.7 percent and never varies more than 4 percent until 2002 (the last date reported), when it drops to 3.3 percent. The U.S. Department of Education has compiled data on the percentage of young adults age 16 to 24 who are not enrolled in a high school program and who have not obtained a diploma or equivalency certificate.[68] These data show that the drop-out rate went from 11.1 percent in 1996 to 10.5 percent in 2002 (last year data is available). This is a decrease of 5.4 percent.

In summary, there is very little data to support progress on Target 12. With the exception of the tuberculosis rate, all indicators regarding the social and health consequences for the general population are in the opposite direction of the goals set in Target 12. For adolescents, there was a 10 percent reduction in the number of emergency room drug episodes but emergency room drug mentions had increased. Many of the changes in risky behaviors of young people correlated with drug use were not in the direction of the goals of Target 12. This also indicates that any reductions in 30-day prevalence among young adolescents have generally not translated into improvements in these risky behaviors among young people.

Targets related to the consequences of drug abuse established in the ONDCP Reauthorization Act of 1998.

5. Reduction of drug-related crime in the United States by 50 percent by December 31, 2003, and achievement of at least 20 percent of such reduction during 1999, 2000,

2001, 2002, and 2003, respectively, including the following:

- Reduction of state and federal unlawful drug trafficking and distribution.

- Reduction of state and federal crimes committed by persons under the influence of unlawful drugs.

- Reduction of state and federal crimes committed for the purpose of obtaining unlawful drugs or obtaining property that is intended to be used for the purchase of unlawful drugs.

- Reduction of drug-related emergency room incidents in the United States (as measured by the Drug Abuse Warning Network), including incidents involving gunshot wounds and automobile accidents in which illicit drugs are identified in the bloodstream of the victim, by 50 percent by December 31, 2003.

As was discussed under Target 11, there is no evidence that drug-related crime has been reduced by 50 percent. On the contrary, crime-related costs of drug abuse and the number of drug-related arrests have increased. For example, the crime-related costs of drug abuse were estimated to be $87.9 billion in 1998 and $107.8 billion in 2002 (last year data were available).[69] From 1998 to 2002 (last year data were available), the total crime index has decreased by 10.8 percent,[70] while the number of incarcerated individuals in state and federal prison has increased by 10.9 percent.[71] From 1998 to 2001 (last year data were available), the number of incarcerated drug offenders in state and federal prison has increased by 10.4 percent.[72] Therefore, any decrease in crime is probably the result of the increasing number of incarcerated individuals. In any case, the target of a 50 percent reduction from 1998 to 2003 will not be achieved.

Three of the four bullets related to this target do not specify a performance measure. However, the data related to the first bullet have already been examined in the discussion of Target 6 through Target 10. There was no evidence on any reduction in drug trafficking and distribution.

The second bullet involves crimes committed by people under the influence of drugs. The only data available comes from the ADAM program that was conducted by the National Institute of Justice. This program was discussed under Target 11, but, to reiterate, the reports on the ADAM program are not consistent in form and content, which makes comparisons over time difficult. In the report regarding 1998 arrestees, 15 of 35 sites had about two-thirds of adult arrestees test positive for at least one illicit drug.[73] In 2003, 25 of the 35 sites reported two-thirds of male adult arrestees tested positive.[74] These data would not be consistent with a reduction in crimes committed by people under the influence of illicit drugs.

There is no direct data to assess the third bullet. With regard to the fourth bullet on emergency room visits, from 1998 to 2002, the total number of emergency room drug abuse episodes increased 27.8 percent. The Drug Abuse Warning Network does not quantify incidents of gunshot wounds and automobile accidents related to drug abuse but does have a category of "accidents/injuries." From 1998 to 2002, there was an increase of 3.6 percent in emergency room drug abuse episodes classified as accidents/injuries.[75]

Conclusion

The activities in the NDCS from 1996 to 2005 have been quite similar. During this 10-year period, $144.57 billion has been spent to implement our NDCS. However, *none* of the target measures have been fully met in either the Clinton or Bush administrations. In fact, the only area in which there has been any progress in the predicted direction has been in the 30-day use patterns of young adolescents, an effect that disappears within 2 to 4 years and cannot be shown to have any impact on the harm caused by drug abuse. With the amount of money that has been spent, the outcomes represent a dismal failure of the NDCS. The situation is a wonderful example of the cliché, "Insanity is doing the same thing over and over again and expecting a different result."

Obviously, the questions are "Why has the NDCS failed?" and "What can be done to change these results?" The remainder of this book will be devoted to these questions.

As a preface to the chapters that address these two questions, it is important to acknowledge the complexity of the problems related to drug use and abuse. Each area, from supply reduction, to prevention, to treatment, has multiple, interrelated factors. For example, our ability to disrupt the supply of drugs from source countries depends upon our relationship with the ruling party of the country. When the Taliban were in control of Afghanistan, the United States had very little influence to control the poppy crop in that country. Antidrug media messages will not be very effective without parental support, and parental support will not be provided in families where there is active alcohol or other drug abuse. Treatment can only work if people with alcohol and other drug problems can access treatment, pay for it, stay in treatment long enough for it to be effective, and have adequate follow-up services. These are only some examples of the complexity of these issues. There are many more. Therefore, simple solutions advocated by anyone, government officials or libertarians, are nonsense.

While acknowledging the complexity of substance abuse problems, it is clear that our current approaches and philosophy have not had the desired effects. Therefore, it does make sense to fully consider alternative conceptualizations and interventions to more effectively reduce the problems of substance abuse. However, as was discussed in Chapter 1, those of us involved in implementing the NDCS are prohibited from discussing certain subjects in an open manner (e.g., legalization of drugs). To answer the questions, "Why has the NDCS failed?" and "What can be done to change these results?" every possible alternative must be openly and fully explored. In the remainder of this book, we will explore controversial topics and examine the utility of incorporating novel approaches into our NDCS.

Three

Legalization, Decriminalization, Harm Reduction

Introduction

The title of this chapter contains the terms that generate the most controversy in this field. Before defining the meaning of legalization, decriminalization, and harm reduction, it is illuminating to read the position of the government as reflected in our NDCS. The first quotation is from the 1999 NDCS and the second from the 2002 NDCS:

> ... small elements at either end of the political spectrum argue that prohibition—and not drugs—create problems. These people offer solutions in various guises, but one of the most trouble-some is the argument that eliminating the prohibition against dangerous drugs would reduce the harm that results from drug abuse. Such legalization proposals are often presented under the guise of "harm reduction."
>
> ... The approach advocated by people who say they favor "harm reduction" when they are really advocating drug legalization would in fact harm Americans.
>
> Some people argue that they are not calling for the legalization of all drugs but only for "soft" drugs. Since many users enter treatment every year for help recovering from chronic abuse of marijuana and similar "soft" drugs, this idea overlooks the danger posed by such drugs. Other people support decriminalization of drugs so that drug use would remain against the law but penalties would be minimal. Illicit drug use would become analogous to minor indiscretions like jay-walking. Still others defend the therapeutic value of specific drugs or the economic viability of a drug-related product.

By making drug use more acceptable, these people argue, society would reduce the harm associated with drug abuse.

The truth is that drug abuse wrecks lives. It is criminal that more money is spent on illegal drugs than on art or higher education, that crack babies are born addicted and in pain, that thousands of adolescents lose their health and future to drugs. Addictive drugs were criminalized because they are harmful; they are not harmful because they are criminalized. The more a product is available and legitimized, the greater will be its use. If drugs were legalized in the U.S., the cost to the individual and society would grow astronomically.

Many harm reduction partisans consider drug use a part of the human condition that will always be with us. While we agree that crime can never be eliminated entirely, no one is arguing that we legalize other harmful activities. At best, harm reduction is a half-way measure, a half-hearted approach that would accept defeat. Increasing help is better than decreasing harm. Pretending that harmful activity will be reduced if we condone it under the law is foolhardy and irresponsible.[1]

"Whether in their undiluted form or in other guises, such as "harm reduction", efforts to legalize drugs represent the ultimate in disastrous social policy. This Administration will oppose them."[2]

Clearly, the same point of view has been expressed by both the Clinton and Bush administrations.

The Meaning of Legalization, Decriminalization, and Harm Reduction

The term "legalization" is not ambiguous. Everyone knows that it is illegal to possess or distribute certain drugs and legalization refers to changing laws to make the possession and/or distribution of these substances legal. However, like most issues in this area, legalization is not as simple as it first appears. For example, medical marijuana laws in some states have made it legal for some people to obtain, possess, use, and/or grow marijuana. While the federal government has maintained that federal laws prohibiting the possession or use of marijuana supersede state laws, states have continued to allow marijuana to be used for medical purposes under the particular state regulations.

The legal status of a drug is determined by the Comprehensive Drug Abuse and Prevention Control Act passed by Congress in 1970 and last amended in 1996. The law classifies drugs of abuse into one of five "schedules." Schedule I drugs have (in the definition of the law) a high potential for abuse, no currently accepted medical use in the United States, and a lack of a safe level of use under medical supervision. Schedule II drugs have high abuse potential and can lead to psychological or physical dependence. However, these drugs have an accepted medical use in treatment. As you might expect, criteria for the progression of the schedules involve the reduction in abuse potential and the probability of dependence and increasing medical uses. Schedule I drugs include heroin, marijuana, LSD, mescaline, peyote, and psilocybin (magic mushrooms). Schedule II drugs include opium, cocaine, and injectable methamphetamine. Schedule III drugs include amphetamine, non injectable methamphetamine, methylphenidate (Ritalin), and opium-based pain medications (e.g., Darvocet, Percodan, OxyContin). Schedule IV drugs include barbiturates and minor tranquilizers (e.g., Valium, Xanax, Ativan) and Schedule V drugs include pain medications with small doses of opium-based drugs.

As you can see, the only drugs that are really "illegal" are marijuana, heroin, and hallucinogens. Other drugs, including cocaine and injectable methamphetamine, are legal but highly regulated.

The categorization of marijuana as a Schedule I drug is certainly controversial. No reputable expert in the field believes that marijuana is more dangerous than cocaine or methamphetamine. The abuse potential of barbiturate (a Schedule IV drug) is far greater than marijuana. A contentious issue is whether marijuana has any medically useful value. This will be discussed in detail in the next chapter.

Finally, it is important to recognize that there are legal, highly addictive, mind-altering drugs available without prescription in the United States. Of course, this refers to alcohol, caffeine, and nicotine.

Therefore, statements in the NDCS about "legalizing drugs" distort important policy issues that should be discussed. Most mind-altering drugs are legal, at least in some circumstances. The policy questions involve regulations on the possession, use, and distribution of these substances and the discussion should involve all mind-altering substances with abuse potential, including alcohol, caffeine, and nicotine.

Decriminalization refers to policies in which drug users are not arrested and charged with a crime. However, there are many variations of decriminalization. The policies may be applied only to specific drugs (e.g., marijuana). Whether or not an arrest is made may be dependent on the amount of the drug in the possession of the person or the circumstances in which it is being used. For example, someone smoking a joint on a street corner would not be arrested but someone driving a car would be. Partial decriminalization policies can involve citations or fines. Under full decriminalization policies, the distribution, production, and/or sale of drugs remain illegal but possession and use of small amounts are not punished.

Harm reduction refers to strategies designed to minimize the negative consequences of drug use. There is an acknowledgment that both legal and illicit drug use is a reality and cannot be totally eliminated. Furthermore, harm-reduction proponents believe that there are differences in the level of safety between methods of using drugs and that drug users should be assisted to use drugs in the safest manner possible. For example, a harm-reduction strategy is needle exchanges, where intravenous drug users are provided with clean, sterile syringes in exchange for used ones.

There are organizations in the United States devoted to harm reduction. For example, the Harm Reduction Coalition ". . . is a nonprofit organization committed to improving the health and well-being of drug users and communities affected by drug-related harm. HRC promotes effective harm reduction services and policies at the national, regional and local levels, through education and training; community organizing; policy advocacy; and publications . . ."[3] On August 19, 2005, this organization sponsored a conference in Salt Lake City: "1st National Conference on Methamphetamine, HIV, and Hepatitis: Science and Response." As a result of the fact that conference planners mistakenly identified the U.S. Department of Health and Human Services as sponsors of the conference, Health and Human Services Secretary Michael Leavitt received a reprimand letter from Congressman Mark Souder, Chairman of the House Subcommittee on Criminal Justice, Drug Policy, and Human Resources that said, "A foundational premise of the so-called "harm reduction" ideology promoted at the HHS-sponsored conference is that we should not be fighting a "war on drugs," but rather limiting drugs' harmful effects. Harm reduction is, in fact, a vehicle drug legalization proponents have hijacked to pave the way to their ultimate objective."[4] Since the organization I directed has activities in Utah, I was contacted by federal officials to determine if we were involved in this conference and to warn us not to participate.

Another organization involved in harm reduction, as well as legalization and decriminalization initiatives is the Drug Policy Alliance. This organization is a merger of the Lindesmith Center and the Drug Policy Foundation. The goals of the Drug Policy Alliance are

- Making marijuana legally available for medical purposes;

- Curtailing drug testing not related to detecting impairment;

- Ending asset forfeiture abuses and restoring constitutional protections against unreasonable searches and seizures;

- Redirecting most government drug-control resources from criminal justice and interdiction to public health and education;

- Supporting public health measures, notably syringe exchange and other harm-reduction programs, to reduce HIV/AIDS, hepatitis, and other infectious diseases;

- Supporting effective, science-based drug education and ending support for ineffective programs;

- Making methadone maintenance and other effective drug treatment more accessible and available;

- Removing obstacles to proper use of opioid and other medications for treatment of pain and terminal disease;

- Repealing mandatory minimum sentences for nonviolent drug offenses and ending incarceration for simple drug possession;

- Ending criminal penalties for marijuana, except those involving distribution of drugs to children;

- Ending invidious discrimination against people with past drug abuse problems or offenses; and

- Ending racially discriminatory drug policies and enforcement measures.[5]

The Drug Policy Alliance is involved in a variety of local, state, and national legislative and policy initiatives. For example, the organization has spearheaded a ballot measure in Oakland, California, to decriminalize marijuana, funded legal actions involving medical marijuana patients, and has helped cities adopt needle exchange programs.

As can be seen, legalization, decriminalization, and harm reduction are not synonymous. The statements in the NDCS and the letter by Congressman Souder attempt to equate these concepts. By doing so, there is an attempt to dissuade people from engaging in a reasonable discussion about the variety of policy issues and strategies incorporated in the terms "legalization, decriminalization, and harm reduction." You may have noticed that the 1999 NDCS attempts to associate harm reduction with totally unrelated, emotional issues such as crack babies.[6]

While it is quite likely that individuals and groups who support very liberal legalization policies also support harm-reduction groups, that does not lead to a conclusion that harm-reduction groups are attempting to legalize drugs. However, that seems to be the position expressed in the NDCS.

An analogy that the Bush administration can relate to will illustrate the faulty logic in equating harm reduction with drug legalization. Individuals and groups who support making Christianity the national religion of the United States also support conservative Republican candidates for office. However, that does not mean that the Republican Party advocates making Christianity the national religion of this country. Similarly, the support of drug legalization advocates for harm-reduction initiatives does not mean that all harm-reduction groups are attempting to legalize drugs.

The History of Drug Policies in the United States[7]

Cocaine, opium, and marijuana have been used by humans for thousands of years. For example, the chewing of coca leaves by South American Indians living in the Andean mountain region dates back to 2500 BC. Marijuana use can be dated back to at least 2737 BC in China and was used as part of religious ceremonies in India thousands of years ago. The ancient Sumerians, Egyptians, and Greeks all have evidence of opium use.

In the more modern era, problems involving opium began in China in the 1600s when the practice of smoking opium became widespread. China outlawed the sale of opium in 1729 because of a growing addiction problem. However, the British were involved with shipping opium to China from India and continued smuggling it in after the ban. Due to the lucrative nature of this endeavor, two Opium Wars were fought between China and Britain from 1839 to 1856. Morphine was first produced from opium in 1803 and codeine followed in 1832. With the development of the hypodermic syringe in 1853, a new method to use these products was created. Opium-derived substances were used during the Civil War, creating many addicts among the soldiers. Opium was also in many patent medicines at the time and many women, particularly in the South, became addicted to these medicines. Heroin was introduced into medicine as a cough suppressant in 1898 by the Bayer Corporation. The Harrison Act of 1914 regulated opium, but heroin was not banned from medical practice in the United States until 1924. Cocaine was a substance in Coca Cola until 1903 and in wines and medicines following that. It was not banned for these uses until the Harrison Act was passed. Cocaine continued to be prescribed for medicinal use into the 1920s. Marijuana was brought to the United States by English settlers and extracts were used by U.S. physicians to produce a tonic for medicinal and recreational purposes. In 1937, the Marijuana Tax Act was passed. This law was modeled after the Harrison Act and prohibited the use of marijuana as an intoxicant and regulated its medicinal use.

In 1951, Congress passed the Boggs Act which created mandatory sentences of 2 years for first offenses and prohibited suspended sentences or probation for subsequent convictions. Harsher penalties were imposed with the passage of the Narcotics Control Act of 1956. This bill dramatically elevated sentences for drug violations, defined marijuana as a narcotic, and set the stage for sentences up to life in prison for possession of marijuana. The Narcotics Control Act of 1956 allowed a death sentence to be imposed for heroin sales to minors.

In an effort to consolidate a number of laws regarding illegal drugs and to extend federal control over hallucinogens and some other drugs, Congress passed The Comprehensive Drug Abuse Prevention and Control Act in 1970. This legislation replaced or updated all other laws on narcotics and other dangerous drugs and is the basis today for our policies on these substances.

Policies and Strategies

In the last 40 years, there have been three major international agreements regarding drug policies. In 1961, the Single Convention on Narcotic Drugs specified controls over opiates, marijuana, and cocaine. In 1971, the Convention on Psychotherapeutic Substances provided controls on drugs that had not been mentioned in the 1961 agreement, including barbiturates, stimulants, and hallucinogens. Finally, the 1988 Convention Against Illegal Traffic in Narcotic Drugs and Psychotropic Substances included criminal penalties for small amounts of illegal substances.[8] These agreements have been described by international drug policy scholars as furthering "... the goals of prohibitionist forces by promoting the ideas that drugs can be controlled through repression, that users can be forced to give up their pleasures, and that the combination of repression and prevention can eventually lead to drug-free societies."[9]

A special, 2004 issue of the Journal of Drug Issues was devoted to drug policy innovations in Central and Western Europe. In a summary article, the role of the United States in influencing the philosophy of these international agreements was described in the following way:

> The evidence presented suggests that the United States and its prohibition allies in the UN have effectively created and sustained a worldwide system of controls that features a strong emphasis on policies that deal with supply-side issues (production, distribution, and sales), and a much weaker commitment to demand-side features (prevention, treatment, and education). Moreover, the entire model is built upon the assumption that the criminal justice approach is both necessary and beneficial in combating the various harms that drugs visit on societies. Alternative models such as public health approaches have been downgraded by prohibition enthusiasts who feel that these methods "coddle" users and serve as dangerous social experiments that can easily lead to the ultimate disaster—the legalization of all substances.[10]

In spite of these international agreements, innovative policies and strategies related to legalization, decriminalization, and harm reduction have been implemented in foreign countries, particularly in Europe. It is not surprising that innovation has taken place outside of the United States, in light of the point of view expressed in the NDCS. Furthermore, the United States has made efforts to dissuade foreign governments from changing prohibitionist drug policies and has strongly criticized those countries that have adopted alternative policies. For example, during the Clinton administration, Drug Czar McCaffrey was an outspoken critic of liberal Dutch drug policies and inaccurately stated publicly that the Dutch had a much higher murder rate than the Americans, attributing the murder rate to these liberal policies.[11] (The Dutch murder rate is actually less than a quarter of the U.S. murder rate.[12]) In response to a Canadian proposal regarding the decriminalization of marijuana, current Drug Czar Walters described the proposal as sending poison to our neighborhood and toxic substances to young people. He also suggested that the result of this policy would be the importation of potent, bioengineered strains of marijuana that would be lead to the crack equivalent of marijuana.[13]

The countries that have adopted innovative strategies regarding drug possession and use, view drug addiction as a public health problem rather than as a criminal matter. In addition, many of these countries have philosophies that preclude government interference in the private behavior of adults if that behavior does not harm others.

It should be noted that, technically, no country which has signed the international treaties could make drugs legal. While it may be splitting hairs, none of the innovations discussed below can be described as "legalization" because the country that implemented such a strategy would be in violation of international agreements.

Decriminalization and depenalization strategies. Most of the strategies in this section are in regard to marijuana. The most well-known innovation regarding marijuana use is in the Netherlands. The Amsterdam coffee shops that sell marijuana are famous and many people believe that marijuana is legal in the Netherlands. However, that is not the case. The production and distribution of marijuana is illegal.[14] There is a formal, written policy of nonenforcement of possession and sale of up to 30 grams of marijuana and tolerance of the sale of small amounts of marijuana in coffee shops. Cities in the Netherlands can determine whether or not to allow coffee shops and most do not. The amount that can be sold to a customer and the quantity of marijuana that is kept on the premises is controlled and a person must be 18 or older to buy. The coffee shop cannot advertise the product and no other drugs can be sold.[15]

Among the European nation states, there has been an increasing trend toward decriminalization and depenalization.[16] For example, in Spain, possession of drugs is illegal but is not an offense unless it is connected to trafficking. Possession of small amounts of illegal drugs is considered self-supply for self-use.[17] In other words, it is illegal to possess drugs in Spain but if you possess a small quantity for your own use, there will be no arrest or penalty. In Italy, possession of small quantities is handled as an administrative rather than as a criminal offense.[18] Belgium treats possession of up to 3 grams of marijuana or cultivation of one plant as criminal offense but the offender is given a simple warning and an on-the-spot fine.[19] In the UK, possession is a criminal offense and the offender could go to court. However, more commonly, the response will be diversion, a warning, or no action.[20]

In Australia, South Australia, the Australian Capital Territory, and the Northern Territory defined a simple cannabis offense as possession of 25 grams or less of marijuana for personal use and cultivation of five or more plants. There is a fine for a simple cannabis offense and, if the fine is paid within 60 days, there is no further action and no conviction is recorded.[21]

In the United States, possession of marijuana has been decriminalized in many states. By 1999, in 15 states, possession of small quantities of marijuana was a misdemeanor with fines but no imprisonment. In another 13 states, the criminal record is expunged after successful completion of education, treatment, and/or community service.[22] However, these state laws conflict with federal policy.

To assess the impact of decriminalization and depenalization strategies, the rates of drug use before and after changes in policies should be compared and drug use rates between jurisdictions with different policies should be examined. Unfortunately, it is difficult to find data that are not complicated by confounding factors. For example, is it important to look at lifetime, 30 day, or daily use? Would the effect of policies impact the extent of youth use, even though no country allows underage drug use? What is the impact of different cultural values between countries on use rates?

In a very thorough review of the literature on marijuana, the impact of prohibition compared to decriminalization on marijuana use is described as follows:

It is clear that prohibition has not eliminated use. It is also clear, however, that criminal sanctions on cannabis use have deterred some individuals from using cannabis, with the most impact on individuals over the age of 30. . . . Neither of these "facts" provides definitive evidence of prohibition's success or failure. We need better data to assess the impact of current policies on individuals' decisions that ideally should come from policy experiments within specific countries and from analyses that account for variations in enforcement and underlying determinants of cannabis use.[23]

With these cautions in mind, there is data on the 30-day use of various drugs by 15- to 16-year-olds from various European countries in 2003.[24] The Netherlands is probably the most inherently interesting because of their liberal policies on marijuana. The percentage of students reporting past month use of marijuana was 13 percent compared to 17 percent among the comparable age group, 10th graders, in the United States in 2003 (see Table 2.5). Among the 35 countries surveyed, the United States had an equivalent or greater percentage of past-month marijuana use than 30 countries. France and the United Kingdom were among the countries with the highest rates of youth marijuana use, and these countries do not have liberal marijuana policies. Switzerland also had a high rate of youth use of marijuana.[25] In that country, the production and use of marijuana is illegal but the industrial production of cannabis (hemp) is not. However, the legally produced cannabis is diverted to illegal use and sold in hemp shops.[26] The Czech Republic and the Isle of Man were the other countries with the highest percentage of youth use. In the Czech Republic, possession of small amounts of marijuana is decriminalized. The Isle of Man is a small, self-governing kingdom in the British Isles and the laws regarding marijuana could not be found. Clearly, these data do not support a hypothesis that liberal marijuana policies result in high rates of marijuana use by youth.

A well-known experiment in decriminalization of injectable drug use was conducted in Switzerland from 1987 to 1992.[27] Due to the difficulty in managing the problems caused by their large addict population, the Swiss decided to ignore drug use as long as it was confined to one location, Platzspitz park. However, this policy resulted in a large increase in the number of injecting drug users in the park, effectively closing the park to the general public. In 1990, 60 Minutes did a story on the park, calling it "Needle Park." With all of the negative publicity, the tolerance policy was ended in 1992. Parenthetically, the rate of drug overdoses increased following the park's closure to injecting drug use.[28]

Harm Reduction Strategies. The rationale for harm reduction strategies has been described in this way:

> Promoters of harm reduction strategies begin with the assumption that drug use can never be eliminated from any society. Consequently, harsh penalties for drug law offenders make little sense as they do not accomplish the desired result and produce harms of their own in the process. Regardless of its obvious appeal for many, a drug-free society is not a realistic goal and should not guide policy in the drug realm. Once one accepts the inevitability of drug

use, questions arise over how the potential harms associated with such use can be reduced and minimized. Harm reduction proponents have established a wide variety of strategies to ameliorate the problems we commonly associate with drug use, and especially with the use of illegal substances. They focus on illegal substances because there are already many harm reduction methods in place for those using legal drugs, such as the widespread distribution of prevention and educational materials, and the existence of a panoply of legal treatment options for those requiring these forms of assistance. Perhaps more importantly, persons using legal drugs are typically left alone and not subjected to harassment, arrest and serious punishments, even though they may be damaging their health and causing those who are close to them a great deal of hardship and misery.[29]

Ironically, some harm reduction strategies are widely used in the United States and actively promoted in the NDCS. For example, opiate substitution therapy (e.g., methadone maintenance) has been used in the treatment of heroin addicts since the mid-1960s.[30] Methadone is a synthetic opiate that eliminates the unpleasant withdrawal from heroin but does not produce heroin's euphoria, allowing the patient to maintain a relatively normal life. Although methadone has traditionally been administered in a limited number of specialized clinics, a revision of federal guidelines now allows qualified providers to be certified to administer methadone. The purpose of this change was to make methadone more accessible for heroin addicts, since, in most cases, a daily dose of methadone is necessary. Since methadone is an addictive substance, the purpose of methadone maintenance therapy is to reduce the harm caused by injecting heroin. More recently, a new opiate, buprenorphine has been approved as a treatment for heroin addiction. Buprenorphine is administered in pill form (methadone is a liquid) by qualified physicians. A daily dose does not seem to be necessary and the withdrawal symptoms are relatively mild. While methadone can be diverted and abused, the pill form of buprenorphine contains another drug that blocks the euphoric properties if the drug is injected. Federal agencies such as the Center for Substance Abuse Treatment and the National Institute on Drug Abuse have actively promoted buprenorphine. In fact, one of the grants I managed had received funds from these agencies to disseminate information about buprenorphine to physicians and other professionals. Again, this is a harm reduction strategy to replace a very harmful, addictive substance (heroin) with a less harmful, addictive substance (buprenorphine).

In Chapter 2, you may recall the many references to "drug courts" and the increasing amount of money devoted to these programs. Drug courts are specialized criminal courts that handle cases involving substance-abusing offenders.

Supervision, drug testing, treatment services, sanctions, and incentives are used to divert these offenders from incarceration.[31] In 1996, there were about 100 drug courts and nearly 1,800 by 2004.[32] The need to reduce prison populations has been a strong motivator to increase the number of drug courts and federal funding has regularly been increased to support these programs. With an emphasis on treatment rather than punishment (although punishment is implemented if offenders don't comply with treatment), drug courts are clearly among the harm reduction strategies. The goal is to reduce the harm that addicts cause society and themselves.

As can be seen, the United States has adopted some harm reduction strategies. Certainly, the statements in the NDCS about harm reduction are referring to other, more controversial initiatives. However, it is important to recognize that harm reduction encompasses a wide range of activities and the U.S. position would be more honest if it acknowledged the government's opposition to only those harm reduction strategies that are politically or philosophically unacceptable to those in power.

A harm reduction strategy that has been implemented in the United States and in many other countries but is opposed by the government is needle exchange programs. In these programs, intravenous drug users can exchange clean syringes for used ones. The purpose is to minimize the spread of HIV, hepatitis, and other blood-borne diseases through infected needles. As of 1998, in the United States, there were 113 needle exchange programs in 80 cities in 38 states.[33] In addition, these programs are common in many other countries. Many needle exchange programs include referrals for treatment and other support services as well as instruction for intravenous drug users on the proper procedures to clean their needles with bleach before use and screening for other diseases such as tuberculosis. The position of the United States is that needle exchange programs imply that intravenous drug use is acceptable. Therefore, the federal government continues to ban federal funding for needle exchange programs, in spite of evidence for their effectiveness in decreasing the transmission of HIV and lack of any evidence that these programs lead to increased drug use.[34]

Heroin distribution programs, another harm reduction strategy, have been successfully operating in Switzerland. As the name implies, these programs involve providing heroin to addicts in controlled doses and in secure settings. In 1994 in Zurich, an experimental program was begun in which one group of addicts received injectable heroin, one group got morphine, and a third group was administered methadone. The participants all had been using heroin for some time and had failed in earlier treatment. They were allowed to choose a dose level that would preclude drug seeking outside the clinic, where they were allowed to inject up to three times a day. They could not take drugs outside of the clinic and were offered support activities regarding employment, health, and family relationships. At the end of 3 years, the heroin group had improved health, employment, and social situations and committed less crimes than before. Based on this evaluation, similar programs were opened in other parts of the country.[35]

Drug consumption rooms are a controversial harm reduction strategy. These programs involve professionally supervised healthcare facilities where drug users can use illegal drugs in a safe, hygienic environment. The drug consumption room is part of a network of services for drug users and is separate from existing services for drug users or for the homeless.[36] The goals of drug consumption rooms include making contact with drug users for the purpose of providing access to social, health, and treatment services; providing a safe, hygienic environment for drug use, particularly for intravenous drug use; reducing the harm of illegal drug use from overdose, the transmission of HIV and hepatitis, and bacterial infections; and minimizing public drug use and its associated problems.[37] As of 2003, there were 72 drug consumption rooms in 39 cities in 4 European countries (Switzerland, the Netherlands, Germany, Spain).[38] To participate, the clients must be dependent on heroin or cocaine. There is a registration process, personalized access cards, and limitations on numbers served. Consumption rooms do not advertise their services and staff cannot help clients inject. However, they can advise clients on safe injecting techniques. Obviously, drug dealing is not allowed. The staff ensures that hygienic and safety procedures are followed. Sterile equipment is provided and the staff observes the administration of drugs.[39]

In 2004, the European Monitoring Centre for Drugs and Drug Addiction reviewed the results of 15 research studies since 2000 on drug consumption rooms.[40] In addition to the possible benefits of reduced high-risk drug use, increased access to treatment and support services, decreases in morbidity and mortality, and reductions in public drug use, the report also focused on the perceived risk of consumption rooms. These risks included increased drug use, initiation of new drug users, delaying treatment due to the perceived acceptance and comfort of drug use, and increases in public disorder by attracting drug users and drug dealers. The results of this review of studies found that consumption rooms do attract street users and older, long-term addicts who have never been in treatment. There was no evidence that consumption rooms recruit new users. Less risky drug use behavior was noted, with no increase in drug use. No conclusion about decreases in communicable diseases could be reached but consumption rooms with adequate access did contribute to a reduction of drug-related deaths. The majority of clients accessed healthcare, social, and treatment services and there was no evidence that clients were more likely to delay treatment. The extent to which consumption rooms reduced public use and community problems was related to their accessibility, operating hours, and capacity. Consumption rooms located near illicit drug markets did not reduce this activity. The report concluded that consumption rooms were most effective when there was community acceptance of this program as part of a comprehensive strategy regarding drug-use problems.[41]

With the rise in ecstasy use in the late 1990s, drug checking became a popular harm reduction strategy, particularly in Europe. As the name implies, drug checking involves testing a substance to determine its contents, with the intent to identify drugs with dangerous adulterants and to prevent the use of these substances. Drug checking has been used to test heroin but came into wider use as a harm reduction strategy when risky imitations of ecstasy came on the market and caused adverse reactions and even death among users. In European countries, warnings about dangerous ecstasy identified by drug checking have been communicated on the Internet.[42] With on-site testing techniques, ecstasy tablets can be tested at raves or other party events with large numbers of young people and the results immediately communicated to the participants. The drug checking service is combined with providing information and education about the risks of drug use and referrals for treatment or other services.[43]

As with many harm-reduction strategies, critics argue that drug checking encourages drug use and creates an environment that is accepting of drug use. Studies in Germany and the Netherlands have not shown that drug checking encourages or increases drug use. These studies have found that unsafe pills were not taken and users became cautious and critical of black market drugs.[44]

The final harm reduction strategy mentioned in this chapter involves regulating the supply of a substance or access to it. This is not the same as the supply reduction activities in the NDCS. For example, limitations on the location and density of retail alcohol outlets have been shown to be related to reductions in alcohol consumption, traffic accidents, and alcohol-related problems.[45] With regard to marijuana, the Dutch try to control access by only allowing sales to adults and by limiting the number of licensed coffee houses. Supply is controlled by specifying the maximum amount of marijuana that can be sold to any customer and the amount of marijuana that can be kept on the premises. As the discussion of decriminalization and depenalization showed, some countries have made an attempt to control marijuana supplies by specifying the number of plants an individual can cultivate without a significant consequence. There are obvious problems with these supply control strategies because the supply of a drug is dependent upon the production and distribution of the substance. In other words, if a country wanted to control the supply of marijuana, it would have to control marijuana growing and/or importation as well as whatever distribution network exists. Theoretically, this could be done within a legalization framework but would be very difficult to accomplish in any decriminalization or depenalization model because the trafficking and distribution of large quantities of drugs remains illegal under decriminalization or depenalization.

Issues Involved with Legalization

The arguments in favor of legalization of drugs are familiar to most people interested in this topic. Drug use by adults is a personal choice and should not be the concern of government, similar to other private behaviors that do not harm others. If drugs were legalized, the production, distribution, and access could be regulated. Tax money could be raised. The criminal element would be taken out of the drug trade. If would be easier to move drug addicts into treatment in a legal, regulated market. Resources currently being used to apprehend and prosecute drug distributors and drug users would be freed up.

As with all of the issues discussed in this chapter, legalization is neither simple nor a panacea for the problems that result from our policies on drugs. First, most European countries differentiate what are called "soft drugs" (e.g., marijuana and hallucinogens) from "hard drugs" (e.g., cocaine, heroin, methamphetamine). Most legalization proposals involve marijuana only. Therefore, all the current problems with the illegality of "hard drugs" would remain. It is only extreme libertarians who are proponents of legalizing all drugs and, frankly, it is difficult to conceptualize a workable system in which adults are legally permitted to purchase and use cocaine, heroin, and methamphetamine. However, that is not an argument for rejecting harm reduction measures involving these drugs.

If we start with the premise that any reasonable model for legalization would only involve marijuana, some of the issues involved with implementing such models can be examined. The first question would be: Would the use of marijuana increase, particularly by young people, if it were legal? According to an analysis of marijuana public health and public policies, the likely answer is "yes."[46] However, the extent of the increase, particularly in regard to heavy, problematic use, would be dependent on price, availability, and access and these variables would be affected by the legalization model that is implemented. For example, marijuana could be distributed through a state-run monopoly, just as alcohol is in some states. This would certainly allow for tight controls on price, availability, and access but may result in more black market marijuana than in other legalization models.

The second major question would involve the social and health costs of legalization. It is unlikely that these costs would be significantly reduced by legalization.[47] As will be seen in the following chapter, marijuana use can have harmful consequences. Increases in traffic accidents and increased health problems as a result of chronic use are unknown but certainly possibilities. A society would have to determine if the unknown negative consequences of legalization would be worth the known consequences of current policy.

The concept of legalization probably raises unrealistic expectations about cost savings in law enforcement. In whatever system is designed, there would be enforcement of this regulated activity and prosecution of those who violate the parameters of the activity. For example, if there is a government monopoly on the sale of marijuana or licensing of distributors, black-marketing would still be illegal. Undoubtedly, there would be regulation of who could grow marijuana, how much could be grown, and the THC content of the marijuana. Underage use would remain illegal. All of this would require the involvement of law enforcement.

The model used to distribute marijuana in a legalized system is another confounding factor. A free market, unregulated system is not likely to be considered seriously by any country. A government monopoly system, in which the government controls the production and distribution of marijuana has already been described. However, a licensing system could also be implemented. This would be analogous to the Netherlands' system which licenses the coffeehouses and regulates them. A similar system could be used to regulate growers. These methods can be used to control the supply and price of marijuana, as well as access to the product. By controlling the price, use of marijuana can probably be manipulated somewhat since increasing the price of alcohol and tobacco by raising excise taxes does result in decreases in alcohol and tobacco use.[48] The problem is that if prices are too high, it becomes more and more lucrative for black marketers to enter the market. Therefore, the goal is to have prices high enough to discourage use (particularly by young people) but low enough to dissuade illegal traffickers and distributors.

Conclusions

The drug policies of the United States have been called "prohibitionist" and "repressive" by harm-reduction proponents, particularly in Europe. The United States is portrayed as having a punishment orientation to drug abuse and addiction, while most European countries are perceived as adopting a treatment orientation. The United States is seen as using the criminal justice system to deal with drug addiction while European countries advocate a public health model that emphasizes the inevitability of drug use, abuse, and addiction. From a public health point of view, interventions are needed to reduce the harm caused by drug use, abuse, and addiction, including various models of treatment.

The United States has taken a hard line against nearly all harm-reduction strategies, seeing them as methods used by legalization proponents to achieve that goal. The United States has been highly critical of foreign countries that propose or adopt decriminalization or harm-reduction programs. These strategies are believed to encourage illicit drug use.

The perception that the United States is totally oriented toward punishing addicts and that Eurpoean countries are totally oriented toward treating addicts is not accurate. The United States is certainly more on the "punishment, criminal justice" end of the continuum than on the "treatment, public health" end. In general, European countries are the opposite. However, some European countries use the criminal justice system to coerce addicts into treatment and arrest and prosecute people for possession of drugs. As has been seen, the United States has adopted and encouraged harm-reduction strategies such as opiate replacement therapies and drug courts. Furthermore, the United States devotes a considerable amount of money to prevention and treatment. A disease concept of addiction and the abstinence model of treatment are the guiding precepts of U.S. treatment policy but, opiate replacement therapy is not an abstinence-based treatment. Therefore, there has been at least some openness to interventions that work but may not fit a favored philosophy.

The point is that extreme positions and hyperbole are not helpful and tend to distort the real issue. The NDCS has failed to achieve its goals. There are strategies that have been used in other places that are worthy of consideration and study. No reasonable person would suggest that the United States immediately implement consumption rooms across the country. However, it is logical to consider a well-designed study of consumption rooms that could be implemented in an urban area with a liberal orientation and a willingness to innovate. Heroin dispensing could be studied in different parts of the country. Various decriminalization and depenalization models could be systematically studied. Clearly, many of the strategies described here would be actively resisted by the majority of people in many communities and, therefore, could not be implemented in those areas.

However, the careful study, planning, and implementation of the strategies described in this chapter in any community requires a willingness on the part of the government to acknowledge the failure of current policies and an openness to creative but politically challenging ideas. So far, those components have been lacking among our policy makers.

Four

How Dangerous Is Marijuana?

Introduction

Marijuana is the most widely used illicit drug. The result of the 2004 National Household Survey showed that nearly 97 million Americans reported using marijuana sometime in their life, nearly 25.5 million had used marijuana in the past year, and over 14.5 million had used this drug in the past month.[1] The number of past month users is nearly seven times the number of past month users of cocaine, the next most widely used illegal drug and more than double the number of past month nonmedical users of prescription drugs.[2] Among young people, age 12–17, 7.6 percent reported using marijuana in the past month and nearly 1 in 5 had used marijuana at some point in their life.[3] Among young adults age 18–25, 16 percent used marijuana in the past month.[4] Over 2 million people used marijuana for the first time in 2004, including over 1.2 million young people.[5]

In terms of illicit drugs, marijuana certainly generates the most controversy. As was seen in Chapter 3, there have been and are decriminalization initiatives domestically and abroad and 11 states have legalized marijuana for medical purposes. There are well-financed efforts to legalize marijuana for personal possession. For example, the Marijuana Policy Project, a nonprofit organization with thousands of members, has sponsored ballot initiatives in Nevada to legalize the possession of small amounts of marijuana, and the activities of the Drug Policy Alliance on marijuana were mentioned in Chapter 3.

ONDCP has devoted significant resources to discouraging marijuana use, especially among young people. In Chapter 2, the Youth Substance Abuse Prevention Initiative begun in 1998 was described, which was primarily designed to reduce youth use of marijuana. In 2002, ONDCP began a Marijuana Initiative.[6] The initiative, which is still going on today, includes youth-and-parenting advertising campaign on television, radio, in magazines, newspapers and online; nonadvertising activities such as partnerships with youth, parent, and health organizations, news media outreach, online resources, outreach to minority audiences, briefings for journalists, outreach to the entertainment industry, classroom resources and activities, and rallies; and resource materials such as a marijuana awareness kit, marijuana posters, downloadable print and broadcast advertising, online content for parents, a PowerPoint presentation for speeches, a video news release, as well as other materials. In addition, ONDCP lists 92 publications on marijuana that are available on its Web site.

Since marijuana is so widely used and since there are continuing efforts to decriminalize or legalize the drug, it is important to evaluate the dangers of marijuana.

The Marijuana Is Dangerous Position

Marijuana is very dangerous, according to ONDCP. In the 2003 NDCS, the effects of marijuana are described in this way:

> . . . marijuana produces withdrawal symptoms and is associated with learning and memory disturbances. Among youth, frequent users of marijuana are four times more likely than non-users to have physically attacked someone during the past six months. Daily marijuana smoking was recently implicated in a five-fold increase of risk for depression and anxiety among females, according to an article in the *British Medical Journal*. . . . Marijuana is the illicit drug most used by pregnant women and women of reproductive age; yet recent research has shown motor, behavioral, and cognitive disturbances in offspring who were exposed to cannabis in the womb. Such disturbances include findings indicative of reduced activity in portions of the brain that regulate emotion and attentiveness. . . . research has now conclusively established that marijuana is addictive. . . . 62 percent [of Americans who meet the criteria for drug treatment] were found to abuse or to be dependent on marijuana . . . These are people with real problems directly traceable to their use of marijuana, including significant health problems, emotional problems, and difficulty in cutting down on use.[7]

In a May 3, 2005, Press Release regarding the relationship between marijuana and serious mental health problems, Drug Czar John Walters said:

> A growing body of evidence now demonstrates that smoking marijuana can increase the risk of serious mental health problems . . . New research being conducted here and abroad illustrates that marijuana use, particularly

during the teen years, can lead to depression, thoughts of suicide, and schizophrenia.[8]

The ONDCP Press Release goes on to say:

A number of prominent studies have recently identified a direct link between marijuana use and increased risk of mental health problems. Recent research makes a stronger case that cannabis smoking itself is a casual agent in psychiatric symptoms, particularly schizophrenia. During the past three years, these studies have strengthened that association and further found that the age when marijuana is first smoked is a crucial risk factor in later development of mental health problems.[9]

In an ONDCP publication called "Marijuana Myths & Facts: The Truth Behind 10 Popular Misperceptions," marijuana is described as "leading to significant health, safety, social, and learning or behavioral problems, especially in young people" with short-term effects including memory loss, distorted perception, thinking and problem-solving difficulties, and anxiety.[10] The publication indicates that marijuana use either causes or is related to cognitive impairment, mental health problems, traffic accidents, use of other illicit drugs, poor academic performance, poor job performance, absenteeism at work, cognitive deficits, lung damage, risky sexual behavior, and violence.[11]

ONDCP has also opposed medical marijuana initiatives. In a March 24, 2003, Press Release regarding proposed legislation in Maryland, Drug Czar Walters said, "Research has not demonstrated that smoked marijuana is safe and effective medicine. Legalizing smoked marijuana under the guise of medicine is scientifically irresponsible and contradictory to our high standards for approval of medications."[12] In a June 6, 2005, Press Release issued after a Supreme Court decision on medical marijuana, Walters stated:

In 1999, the Institute of Medicine (IOM) published a review of the available scientific evidence in an effort to assess the potential health benefits of marijuana and its constituent cannabinoids. The review concluded that smoking marijuana is not recommended for any long-term medical use, and a subsequent IOM report declared, "marijuana is not a modern medicine."[13, 14]

The Marijuana Is Not Dangerous Position

Marijuana is not dangerous, according to organizations such as the National Organization for the Reform of Marijuana Laws (NORML). As evidence, they cite an editorial from a British medical journal that begins, "The smoking of cannabis, even long term, is not harmful to health."[15] The NORML Web site also contains information from a 1997 book on marijuana myths and facts, published by the Lindesmith Center, a policy reform institute.[16] According to this source, marijuana is not physically addicting and only a very small minority of marijuana users develop a dependency on the drug. Most of these individuals are able to discontinue their use without difficulty, experiencing only mild withdrawal. There is no causal relationship between marijuana use and the use of other drugs. Studies of long-term, high-dosage use of marijuana have not found any brain damage in humans as a result of this level of use. According to this analysis, adult marijuana users who work earn higher wages than nonusers and college student marijuana users earn the same grades as nonusers. They acknowledge that heavy use by high school students is associated with school failure but contend that the school failure precedes the marijuana use. Short-term memory is impacted while intoxicated but lasts only as long as the person is intoxicated. They dispute the contention that there is any convincing evidence that long-term marijuana use permanently impacts memory or other cognitive processes. According to this report, there is no evidence that marijuana causes mental illness, although psychological distress can be an adverse acute effect and large doses can result in a temporary toxic psychosis, usually as a result of ingesting marijuana. The studies cited indicate that marijuana reduces rather than increases aggression. This report indicates that prenatal marijuana exposure has no consistent adverse effect on physical, developmental, or cognitive deficits in children. The authors acknowledge that an increased risk of lung cancer from smoking marijuana cannot be ruled out but that emphysema is not likely to result from smoking marijuana. Moderate marijuana smoking is described as posing only minimal danger to the respiratory system. While marijuana may impact driving, most people drive more carefully while intoxicated with marijuana and traffic accidents are usually the result of a combination of marijuana and alcohol. Marijuana has definite medical uses, including reducing the nausea from chemotherapy, stimulating appetite in AIDS patients, reducing intraocular pressure in people with glaucoma, and reducing muscle spasticity in people with neurological disorders. Smoked marijuana is described as more effective for these conditions than the commercially prepared medication containing THC, the major active ingredient in marijuana.

Clearly, the "facts" presented by ONDCP and NORML are in conflict. It would be very difficult for the average person or for most professionals to separate scientific evidence from propaganda. And, it is very important to disseminate accurate information about the risks of marijuana use and any adverse effects, given the large number of young people using this drug. If the information regarding the dangers of marijuana is exaggerated, misrepresented, or falsified, it will be in conflict with the experience of these users and their peers and make it unlikely that they will seriously attend to information about the dangers of any drugs. If the actual dangers of marijuana are minimized or distorted, there is less chance that current users will be influenced to modify their behavior or new users dissuaded from initiating use. What is the truth about the dangers of marijuana?

Objective Information on Marijuana

There are two primary sources for the information in this section. In 1998, ONDCP supported a study by the National Academy of Sciences' Institute of Medicine (IOM) on marijuana's potential benefits and harms. In one of the quotes from Drug Czar John Walters in an earlier section of this chapter, he refers to a result from this study. The IOM report is one source for the information reviewed here. [17] The second source is a book titled *Cannabis Use and Dependence: Public Health and Public Policy* (Cannabis Book).[18] The authors are from the University of Queensland (Australia) and the RAND Corporation's Drug Policy Research Center, a well-respected organization that receives a lot of federal grant money in the substance abuse area. The Cannabis Book contains an impressive review of literature on all aspects of marijuana use, effects, and policy. In a review appearing in a professional journal, this book was described as ". . . the most comprehensive and honest attempt to improve the quality of the public policy debate on cannabis."[19] While it is probably not possible for any source to be completely objective, these documents seem to be very balanced and no discernable bias could be detected.

The mission of the IOM was to assess the possible medical benefits of marijuana compared to the harms of the drug. Therefore, the IOM report did not consider as many aspects of marijuana use as did the Cannabis Book, and the Cannabis Book relied on the IOM report for most of the information on the potential medical benefits of marijuana. The results of the IOM report will be reviewed first and then the conclusions in the Cannabis Book will be summarized.

The IOM report describes the effect of THC, the primary psychoactive ingredient in marijuana; cannabinoids, which are the compounds related to THC; and marijuana, the unpurified plant substances. The IOM report studied the effects of isolated cannabioids and concluded that they have a natural role in pain modulation, control of movement, and memory. The role on cannabioids in the immune system was unclear and the report concluded that the brain develops tolerance to cannabioids. While animal research demonstrated dependence on cannabioids, the potential for dependence was seen as occurring under a more narrow range of conditions than for drugs such as minor tranquilizers, opiates, cocaine, or nicotine. Withdrawal symptoms were observed in animal studies but were mild compared to drugs such as minor tranquilizers or opiates.

The IOM report also reviewed research on the efficacy of cannabinoid drugs. The conclusion was that there was scientific evidence for the potential therapeutic value of THC for pain relief, nausea and vomiting control, and appetite stimulation. However, the IOM report also indicated that smoking marijuana was an imprecise method to deliver THC and produced harmful substances through smoking. The report also discussed the psychological effects of marijuana, such as anxiety reduction, sedation, and euphoria. It was determined that these psychological effects can influence the therapeutic effects in potentially beneficial or harmful ways. For example, some older patients reported that the psychological effects were disturbing. For patients with AIDS wasting syndrome, the combination of appetite stimulation with the psychological effects of anxiety reduction, sedation, and euphoria could be beneficial.

The IOM report also examined the risks associated with the medical use of marijuana. With the exception of the harms associated with smoking, the detrimental effects of marijuana were seen as being within the range that is tolerated for other medications. The acute effects included diminished psychomotor performance, which could impact driving or the operation of dangerous equipment. A small number of marijuana users experienced unpleasant feelings from the drug. The acute effects on the immune system could not be firmly established but, if such effects exist, were not severe enough to rule out the use of marijuana for medicinal purposes. With regard to chronic effects, the conclusion was that marijuana smoke is associated with increased risk of cancer, lung damage, and poor pregnancy outcomes. There was no convincing evidence that marijuana smoke does or does not cause respiratory cancer.

Another chronic effect of marijuana studied in the IOM report involved dependence and withdrawal. The conclusion was that while few marijuana users develop dependence on the psychoactive effects, some do, and the risk factors for the development of dependence are similar to other drugs. A withdrawal syndrome was identified, consisting of restlessness, irritability, minor agitation, difficulty sleeping, nausea, and cramping, although the symptoms were judged to be mild and short.

The IOM report discussed the issue of marijuana as a "gateway" drug. That is, does marijuana use lead to the use of other drugs? The investigators found no evidence that there is any inherent characteristic of marijuana that could be linked in a causal manner to the subsequent use of other drugs. There certainly is a progression for most drug users from tobacco to alcohol to marijuana and then to other drugs. In this way, marijuana is a "gateway" to other drugs but tobacco and alcohol are the first "gateways" in this progression. There was also no evidence that the use of marijuana for medicinal purposes would increase the use of marijuana among the general population, assuming medical marijuana was regulated in the same manner as other medications with the potential for abuse.

The IOM report also contains a detailed discussion of the risk/benefit ratio of smoking marijuana for medicinal purposes. Since Drug Czar Walters has used this section of the IOM report to argue against medical marijuana, it is important to read the exact language on this issue in the report:

> Because of the health risks associated with smoking, smoked marijuana should generally not be recommended for long-term medical use. Nonetheless, for certain patients, such as the terminally ill or those with debilitating symptoms, the long-term risks are not of great concern. Further, despite the legal, social, and health problems associated with smoking marijuana, it is widely used by certain patient groups ... The goal of clinical trials of smoked marijuana would not be to develop marijuana as a licensed drug but rather to serve as a first step toward the possible development of nonsmoked rapid-onset cannabinoid delivery systems. However, it will likely be many years before a safe and effective cannabinoid delivery system, such as an inhaler, is available for patients. In the meantime there are patients with debilitating symptoms for whom smoked marijuana might provide relief. The use of smoked marijuana for those patients should weigh both the expected efficacy of marijuana and ethical issues in patient care, including providing information about the known and suspected risks of smoked marijuana use ... Until a nonsmoked rapid-onset cannabinoid drug delivery system becomes available, we acknowledge that there is no clear alternative for people suffering from *chronic* conditions that might be relieved by smoking marijuana, such as pain or AIDS wasting. [italics in original][20]

You may recall that, in referring to the IOM study, Drug Czar Walters said the report concluded that smoked marijuana did not have *any* long-term medical use. That would appear to be a misrepresentation of the conclusions in this report. This distortion is also printed in the ONDCP publication *Myths & Facts: The Truth Behind 10 Popular Misperceptions*: "In 1999, the Institute of Medicine (IOM) published a review of the available scientific evidence in an effort to assess the potential health benefits of marijuana and its constituent cannabinoids. The review concluded that smoking marijuana is not recommended for any long-term medical use, and a subsequent IOM report declared, 'marijuana is not a modern medicine.'"[21]

In spite of the federal government's position on medical uses of marijuana, 11 states have adopted "medical marijuana" laws. Only three of these states have enacted these laws through the legislative process. The other eight have been the result of ballot initiatives.[22]

The Cannabis Book is a very thorough review of scientific literature on all aspects of marijuana use, including the pharmacology, use patterns, benefits of marijuana, acute and chronic effects from marijuana on psychological and physical health, the impact on adolescents, and the effect of policy decisions. The focus here will be to summarize the conclusions regarding the danger or harmful effects of marijuana.

For those areas that overlap with the IOM report, there is consistent agreement. That would be expected since both works reviewed the same scientific literature. However, the Cannabis Book was published 4 years after the IOM report, so the Cannabis Book did have the benefit of reviewing more sources.

Acute physical and psychological effects. Marijuana intoxication has an adverse effect on attention span, short-term memory, and psychomotor performance. Anxiety and panic attacks can occur, primarily in new users who are not familiar with marijuana's effects. At very high doses, some people experience delusions and hallucinations. There are no cases of fatal marijuana poisoning and humans are very unlikely to be able to ingest a fatal dose. The effect of marijuana intoxication impairs motor and cognitive abilities necessary to safely drive a car or operate machinery. The extent to which marijuana is involved in auto accidents is unclear. Many motorists intoxicated with marijuana drive more slowly and carefully and take fewer risks. However, there is an increased risk of accidents after using marijuana, but marijuana alone does not appear to contribute a great deal to accidents. Marijuana in combination with alcohol does.

Physical Effects of Chronic Use. Marijuana smoke contains carcinogens. However, because of nondefinitive or conflicting results, additional research on the association between smoking marijuana and certain cancers should be conducted. There is no evidence that the rate of infectious diseases is increased among heavy marijuana users. However, with very high doses of marijuana, animal studies have shown immune system impairment, reduced resistance to infection, and compromises in the immune defense system in the lungs. Studies of HIV patients who use marijuana have not produced evidence of an accelerated progression to AIDS. The use of marijuana during pregnancy is associated with small birthweight but not with an increased risk of birth defects. Similar, but smaller, behavioral and developmental effects resulting from maternal tobacco use have been seen in studies of infants prenatally exposed to marijuana. Animal studies have demonstrated disruption in the reproduction system from chronic administration of THC. However, no definitive research has been conducted on the impact of heavy marijuana use on the reproductive systems of humans. The changes in heart rate and blood pressure from marijuana use are not likely to have an adverse impact on healthy adults but could be harmful to those with hypertension, at high risk for strokes, or with clogged heart arteries. Because marijuana smoke contains many of the same carcinogens found in tobacco smoke, it is likely that marijuana smoking increases the risk of respiratory cancers, especially if used in combination with tobacco. The regular use of smoked marijuana impairs the functioning of the airways and can cause chronic bronchitis. There is no evidence of any adverse effect of marijuana on the liver or gastrointestinal system.

Psychological Effects of Chronic Use. In the late 1960s, an amotivational syndrome was described in which young marijuana users were seen as apathetic, withdrawn, lethargic, and unmotivated. However, there is no evidence of a unique syndrome with these symptoms that is attributable to marijuana use. These symptoms are more likely the result of marijuana dependence. Clearly, heavy marijuana use can lead to dependence on the drug, characterized by a combination of social, legal, financial, family, educational, and occupational problems; withdrawal symptoms when drug use is discontinued; and difficulty in controlling the use of marijuana in spite of the intention to do so. The rate of abuse and dependence problems from marijuana is lower than that of alcohol and more people with marijuana problems are able to discontinue their use without treatment than is found with other addicting substances. Daily, long-term use of marijuana may adversely impact memory, attention, and the integration of complex information in subtle ways. However, there does not seem to be any severe impairment of cognitive functioning. There is still some uncertainty regarding whether all the impairments are reversible after a long period of abstinence.

ONDCP has devoted a lot of attention recently to the relationship between marijuana and mental health through a 2005 publication, "The Link Between Marijuana and Mental Illness: A Survey of Recent Research."[23] Some of the statements from the press release on this publication were provided earlier in this chapter. The Cannabis Book analysis supports the contention that there is a relationship between heavy marijuana use and mental health problems. However, the interpretation of the nature of this relationship is different than that of ONDCP. For example, the Cannabis Book does conclude that young people who use marijuana are at high risk for mental health problems. Some of this is explained by the fact that these young people were at high risk for mental health problems before they began to use marijuana. In addition, young people who begin using marijuana at a young age are more likely to affiliate with delinquent and/or drug using peers, which increases their risk for a variety of problems. Finally, it should be noted that the early first use of tobacco and alcohol is also associated with later mental health problems. Therefore, the likely mediating variables that explain the association between marijuana and mental health problems involve the predisposing characteristics of the user and the lifestyle associated with illicit drug use.

There is evidence that marijuana can precipitate psychosis in people who are vulnerable to developing psychotic disorders. In other words, some people will develop schizophrenia or another psychotic disorder if the proper environmental conditions are present (e.g., trauma). The heavy use of marijuana may be one of those environmental factors. In spite of the implication that marijuana can cause schizophrenia, this does not seem likely. During the years when marijuana use has increased among adults, the incidence of schizophrenia has been stable or decreased.

Similarly, there is an association between adolescent marijuana use and non-completion of high school, involvement in drug-related crime, early pregnancy, and divorce. Again, the characteristics of the adolescent marijuana user seem to be the factors that explain these associations. However, there is little doubt that the early use of marijuana is among the risk factors that are associated with a variety of adolescent problems.

Comparison between alcohol and marijuana. It can be difficult to evaluate the relative danger of marijuana without a comparison to alcohol. When a summary of the dangers of marijuana is reviewed, the drug may sound very damaging. But, most people are not aware of all of the dangers of alcohol and a review of the results of alcohol abuse may (or may not) have an impact on a person's assessment of the danger of marijuana. Clearly, alcohol is legal for adults over 21 to use and marijuana is not. Therefore, marijuana is inherently more dangerous to possess than alcohol. However, this analysis, conducted in the Cannabis Book, involves the acute and chronic effects of these substances.

Alcohol and marijuana share some common effects from acute intoxication, including impaired psychomotor coordination and cognitive functioning. The impact of acute alcohol intoxication on the operation of motor vehicles is well known and the consequences can be extremely damaging. The evidence regarding marijuana is less compelling, although the combination of alcohol and marijuana is quite dangerous. Impulse control and judgment are impacted from intoxication with either substance. Alcohol intoxication is strongly associated with aggression and violence and may be a factor in suicide. Marijuana is not associated with aggression and violence. Some studies have suggested a relationship to suicide while others have not. Alcohol consumption during pregnancy can result in fetal alcohol syndrome. Marijuana consumption during pregnancy is associated with low birth weight but not with birth defects. Acute alcohol overdose can cause death by asphyxiation, alcohol poisoning, inflammation of the heart muscles, and heart attack. No human fatalities from marijuana overdose have occurred.

Chronic alcohol and marijuana use can lead to dependence on these substances. The withdrawal symptoms from alcohol can be dangerous and should be monitored in detoxification facilities. The withdrawal from marijuana is milder and not physically dangerous. About 15 percent of those who ever use alcohol become dependent on it, while about 10 percent of marijuana users become dependent. More marijuana than alcohol dependent individuals spontaneously discontinue their use (i.e., quit without treatment).

Chronic alcohol use is a cause of liver cirrhosis, gastritis, high blood pressure, stroke, irregular heartbeat, weakened heart muscles, pancreatitis, and malfunction of the peripheral nerves and a contributing cause to cancers in the digestive system and breasts. There is evidence that the moderate use of some forms of alcohol may have a role in the prevention of heart disease. Moderate marijuana use has no known health benefits. Chronic marijuana use may cause cancers in the aerodigestive tract and increase the risk for respiratory diseases. Chronic marijuana use probably causes subtle impairment in cognitive functioning but it is unclear if this is permanent or dissipates following prolonged abstinence. Chronic, heavy alcohol use can cause severe brain damage. Psychosis is related to both alcohol and marijuana use. In chronic alcohol users, intoxication or withdrawal can produce psychotic symptoms. Chronic use of marijuana may produce psychotic symptoms or precipitate psychosis in vulnerable individuals. Occupational and educational performance is adversely impacted by chronic marijuana or alcohol use, although the effects on occupational functioning seem to be more severe with alcohol.

Treatment admissions and emergency room visits. Another way to assess the danger of marijuana is to examine the number of people treated for marijuana abuse or dependence and the number of emergency room episodes in which marijuana is a factor. According to information from federal government, admissions to treatment in which the patient reported marijuana was the primary substance of abuse more than doubled from 1993 to 2003.[24] In 1993, 7 percent of all admissions mentioned marijuana as the primary drug of choice while 16 percent reported this in 2003. However, most of this increase was driven by referrals from the criminal justice system. In 1993, 48 percent of the marijuana treatment admissions were referred from the criminal justice system while this rate increased to 57 percent in 2003.[25] Therefore, it is not possible to tell if the increase in treatment admissions is due to law enforcement changes (i.e., drug courts) or actual increases in marijuana dependence.

According to the Drug Abuse Warning Network, there were 627,923 emergency room visits related to drugs in the last half of 2003 and 12.7 percent of these visits included marijuana as a drug that either induced or related to the emergency room visit.[26] In 4.5 percent of these cases, the emergency room visit involved a suicide attempt, 10.9 percent involved a desire for detoxification, and nearly all of the rest (84 percent) were categorized as "other." In comparison, cocaine accounted for 20.1 percent of the drug-related emergency room visits. Of these, 3.6 percent were related to a suicide attempt, 23.0 percent to a desire for detoxification, and

72.9 percent were "other." Heroin was involved in 7.6 percent of the emergency room visits and methamphetamine was mentioned in 4 percent of the cases. Therefore, marijuana was mentioned more often than any other illicit drug except cocaine. Alcohol in combination with another drug was involved in 19 percent of the emergency room visits. Of these, 26 percent involved a suicide attempt, 33 percent detoxification, 1 percent adverse reactions, 22 percent overmedication, 59 percent malicious poisoning, and 28 percent "other."[27]

Does marijuana use lead to other drug use? This is frequently referred to as the "gateway" theory. That is, the use of marijuana is a "gateway" to the use of other drugs. The IOM report did not find any evidence that there was something inherent in marijuana that caused a person to use other drugs. The Cannabis Book examined this issue in great detail. While there is no disputing the fact that marijuana users are more likely than nonmarijuana users to use other drugs and that the earlier the age of first use of marijuana, the more likely the individual is to use other drugs, the relationship between these facts and the "gateway" theory is controversial. As the IOM study stated and the Cannabis Book validates, there is no evidence that marijuana has some pharmacological property that would cause a user to crave other drugs. The most likely explanations for the relationships between marijuana and other drug use involve the characteristics of marijuana users and peer and environmental influences. Those individuals who use marijuana at an early age and/or use marijuana heavily may have genetic, personality, and attitudinal characteristics that predispose them to use mind-altering substances. Since marijuana is the most widely available illicit drug and is perceived as the least harmful illicit drug, it makes sense that this drug would be used first. As was previously stated, the fact that tobacco and alcohol use almost always precedes marijuana use is further evidence that the most widely available substance will be used first. Furthermore, those young people who use marijuana are affiliating with peers who also use marijuana, who are accepting of illicit drug use, who generally support the experimentation of other drugs, and who have some knowledge of how to secure illicit drugs. These generalizations do not always fit, since there are certainly peer groups who use marijuana but who disapprove of the use of other drugs and all marijuana users do not progress to the use of other drugs. In fact, most do not. However, it is not difficult to conceptualize a 13-year-old who begins to use marijuana as associating with a peer group which is accepting of drug use in general, while an 18-year-old who first uses marijuana may be involved in a peer group whose illicit drug use is limited to marijuana. The 13-year-old initiate is much more likely to be rebellious, risk-taking, and unconventional than the 18-year-old initiate. This would explain the relationship between age of first use of marijuana and the use of other drugs.

Barriers to Research

The IOM report contained six recommendations. Five of these recommendations involved research, including clinical trials involving marijuana. In a 2004 editorial in Scientific American, the editors stated:

> . . . regulations and attitudes thwart legitimate research with marijuana. Indeed, American biomedical researchers can more easily acquire and investigate cocaine. Marijuana is classified as a so-called Schedule I drug, alongside LSD and heroin. As such, it is defined as potentially addictive and having no medical use, which under the circumstances becomes a self-fulfilling prophecy. Any researcher attempting to study marijuana must obtain it through the National Institute on Drug Abuse (NIDA). The U.S. research crop, grown at a single facility, is regarded as less potent—and therefore less medicinally interesting—than the marijuana often easily available on the street. Thus, the legal supply is a poor vehicle for studying the approximately 60 cannabinoids that might have medical applications. The system has unintended, almost comic, consequences. For example, it has created a market for research marijuana, with "buyers" trading journal co-authorships to "sellers" who already have a marijuana stockpile or license. The government may also have a stake in a certain kind of result. One scientist tells of a research grant application to study marijuana's potential medical benefits. NIDA turned it down. The scientist rewrote the grant to emphasize finding marijuana's negative effects. The study was funded.[28]

There is always room for an intellectually honest disagreement about any subject, and marijuana, especially the medical uses for the drug, is no exception. However, the barriers to research that are described in this editorial are inexcusable. Marijuana may have no medical benefits that justify its use or it may have some medical benefits that can relieve the pain and suffering of seriously ill people. However, without the proper research, conclusions are impossible to reach. Logically, it would be in the government's interest to facilitate research since federal officials, especially the Drug Czars, seem to be very secure in their position on marijuana. Therefore, the barriers to research are puzzling and lead to suspicions that federal officials are afraid the results that would come from solid research would be contrary to their beliefs. This suspicion is reinforced by the way the results and recommendations of the IOM report have been largely ignored by federal officials. The only reference to the IOM report in the ONDCP publication, *Myths & Facts: The Truth Behind 10 Popular Misperceptions* is the misrepresentation of the IOM's conclusion about the medical use of smoked marijuana.

Marijuana is a mind-altering, potentially addictive drug.

Conclusions

The title of this chapter posed a question, "How dangerous is marijuana?" ONDCP's position is that marijuana is very dangerous. Marijuana advocacy groups like NORML claim that marijuana is not dangerous at all. Both sides claim that the scientific evidence supports their position. Therefore, objective reviews of the research literature were examined to determine the answer to the question about the danger of marijuana and to assess the accuracy of the claims on each side of this argument.

Clearly, both sides pick and choose the information *concl.* that supports their position. The objective information leads to these conclusions: Marijuana is a mind-altering, potentially addictive drug. Some acute and chronic effects can be damaging. There are probably some medical uses for marijuana. Marijuana is not nearly as dangerous acutely or chronically as alcohol. More research is needed to determine the potential benefits and harms of marijuana.

NORML's use of the "scientific" information is understandable. The mission of the group is to legalize marijuana. The organization is privately funded and, therefore, has no obligation to the public. The group can selectively focus on information that supports its point of view, take information out of context, ignore research that contradicts its position, or misrepresent the conclusions of others. In other words, NORML is no different than any other private advocacy group that wants to influence public policy.

On the other hand, ONDCP is part of the U.S. government. It is funded with public dollars and should be held to a high standard of scrutiny regarding publications and public statements. It should not be acceptable for a government agency to selectively use data to support a position and ignore data that contradicts its position.

Through both the Clinton and Bush administrations, ONDCP has used unethical methods to portray marijuana in a negative manner. As was seen with Drug Czar Walters' statement about the IOM report conclusion on the medical use of smoked marijuana, information was changed and taken out of context to completely alter the meaning. In the 2003 NDCS, selective research is cited to support negative effects of marijuana but research that does not support these negative effects is ignored. ONDCP statements and publications often use correlational events to imply that marijuana causes these events. For example, the 2003 NDCS mentions that young marijuana users are four times more likely than nonusers to have physically attacked someone in the past 6 months. The intent of such a statement is to create the impression that marijuana causes violence. As was seen in the objective assessment of research, there is no evidence of such a relationship. ONDCP has diligently tried to establish a cause and effect relationship between marijuana use and mental health problems, in spite of the alternative, more plausible explanations for the relationship between heavy marijuana use and mental health problems. There is a consistent effort to imply that the use of marijuana leads to the use of other drugs, when again, there are other explanations to explain the relationship between marijuana and the use of other drugs.

While these strategies are not excusable, they are understandable. Marijuana is the illicit drug most used by young people (as well as adults) and no logical person believes that it is good for adolescents to use drugs. Furthermore, if ONDCP is going to show any impact on illicit drug use, it is likely to be in the use of marijuana, simply because of the number of young people who use it. Therefore, since ONDCP certainly wants to show that their efforts are having an impact on illicit drug use, it makes sense to focus on marijuana. In spite of evidence that scare tactics do not dissuade young people from using drugs, perhaps ONDCP believes that making marijuana sound as bad as possible will influence young people to avoid using this drug. At the very least, parents may be persuaded to be more concerned with the possible use of marijuana by their children. Of course, some very suspicious people believe that ONDCP's real agenda is to maintain a focus on marijuana so that attention is not directed toward the drug that causes the most harm among young people, alcohol.

No matter what the motivations of ONDCP are, the methods are inappropriate and not likely to be successful. As was seen in Chapter 2, all of the efforts to demonize marijuana have not any demonstrable effect. While the 30-day use of marijuana has gone down among school-aged youth in the last 10 years, it has gone up among college students and young adults in the last nine years (see Table 2.5). The daily use of marijuana has risen dramatically among college students and young adults (see Table 2.8) as has the 30-day use of illicit drugs other than marijuana (see Table 2.4). Therefore, even if some young people are delaying their use of marijuana until they are older, what good has this done?

The most inexplicable and illogical position of ONDCP involves the medicinal use of marijuana. It is frankly appalling that the director of ONDCP, a cabinet-level government official, would misrepresent the findings in the IOM report regarding the use of smoked marijuana for persons with debilitating and/or terminal illnesses. That this was done to protect a political position opposing any use of medical marijuana makes it even worse. It makes no sense to argue that prescribing marijuana for medical purposes will lead to legalization or wider distribution to young people. Opiate-based drugs are prescribed for pain management but can also be abused and lead to addiction. That's why it requires a physician's prescription to get them. That doesn't prevent these drugs from being abused but it does provide regulatory controls on their use. Minor tranquilizers (e.g., Ativan, Valium, Xanax) are prescribed for a variety of "medical" purposes, most of which involve helping people feel better when they are anxious or stressed. They are addictive and can be abused. No one is advocating for the sale of opiate-based pain medications or minor tranquilizers over-the-counter in drug stores. Why would physician-prescribed marijuana lead to this? In addition, the proposed medical uses of marijuana involve very serious medical conditions, not helping the modern American cope with everyday stress as is the case with many of the prescriptions for minor tranquilizers. The hypocrisy in this situation is impressive.

However, there should be no misunderstanding about this: Marijuana is not a harmless substance. No mind-altering, potentially addictive substance is harmless. The information in the IOM report and the Cannabis Book was compelling about the physical and psychological dangers of marijuana. The issue does not revolve around whether or not the use of marijuana can lead to negative consequences. Rather, it seems to be ONDCP's obsession with marijuana, the relentless attempts to twist the objective information on this drug to fit its position, and its obstinate resistance to scientifically evaluating any medical benefits to marijuana.

Five

Why Doesn't the NDCS Focus on Underage Drinking?

Introduction

The simple answer to the question in the title of this chapter is that alcohol is not included in ONDCP's mandate from Congress. As you will recall from Chapter 1, ONDCP was started by the passage of the Anti-Drug Abuse Act of 1988. ONDCP has been reauthorized by Congress several times, most recently in 1998. It was scheduled to be reauthorized in 2003 but that legislation never made it out of committee. There was another reauthorization bill in Congress in the fall of 2005 that has not been acted on at the time this is being written (June 2006). There is no language in any previous bill or the current bill that provides ONDCP with the Congressional authorization to deal with alcohol.

However, you will recall from Chapter 2 that Barry McCaffrey, Drug Czar in the Clinton administration, did include a target about youth alcohol and tobacco use in the 1999 NDCS. Furthermore, there are some federal initiatives in agencies that primarily have functions under the auspices of ONDCP (e.g., Substance Abuse and Mental Health Services Administration) which involve underage drinking. Therefore, it is reasonable to ask why more is not being done.

ONDCP has clearly not advocated for increasing their involvement in underage drinking prevention. In 1999, an amendment was introduced in Congress to change the authorizing legislation for ONDCP to allow underage drinking prevention messages in the national antidrug media campaign. Drug Czar McCaffrey, along with the alcohol industry, opposed the amendment and it was defeated.[1] The following year, the National Media Campaign to Prevent Underage Drinking Act of 2000 was introduced to authorize a separate media campaign to prevent and reduce underage drinking. That legislation was stalled by the alcohol industry pending the completion of a study of underage drinking by the National Academy of Sciences.[2] Although that study has been completed (and will be discussed later in the chapter), the legislation was never acted on.

Because of pressure from the alcohol industry, neither the federal administration (represented by ONDCP) nor Congress is interested in having ONDCP focus on alcohol. In this chapter, there will be a discussion of how this policy is illogical, based on the harm caused by underage drinking and the relationship of youth alcohol and illicit drug use.

Alcohol Use By Adults

Before discussing underage drinking, it is important to understand what alcohol is and how it is used and abused by adults. Alcohol is a mind-altering drug, just like illicit drugs. Since it is a legal drug, many people tend to think it is different. That is the reason why the phrase "alcohol and other drugs" is often used in this book. Otherwise, if the term "drugs" was used, many people would think that alcohol was not part of the discussion. Theoretically, it would be great if everyone understood that mind-altering drugs include alcohol.

Most adults use alcohol. Table 5.1 shows the 2004 National Household Survey of the percentages of adults age 18–25 and 26 and older who drink alcohol, binge drink (5 or more drinks at one sitting), or have an alcohol abuse or dependence disorder.[3]

The majority of adults drink alcohol at least once a month. A very large number of adults binge drink at least monthly. Far more adults have alcohol problems than illicit drug problems. It is also worth noting that the rates of binge drinking, as well as alcohol abuse and alcohol dependency, fall dramatically as people get older. This is similar to what was observed with regard to illicit drug use. There is a "maturing out" of heavy alcohol use. In addition, people with alcohol abuse or dependency problems may get treatment and stop drinking and some may die.

In Chapter 4, the dangers of alcohol and marijuana were compared. Clearly, alcohol is more damaging acutely and chronically than this illegal drug. In Chapter 1, the costs of alcohol and drug abuse were compared (see Table 1.2). The economic costs of alcohol abuse were nearly double those of drug abuse. If the crime-related costs were removed (since drugs are illegal and alcohol is not), the economic costs of alcohol abuse would be more than four times that of drug abuse. Similarly, there are more than four times the number of alcohol-related deaths as those deaths caused by illegal drug abuse.

Given this information on alcohol abuse and the harm resulting from it, why limit this discussion to underage drinking? First, the NDCS is about the illicit and illegal use of drugs. Even with the knowledge that alcohol is a drug, alcohol use

Table 5.1

Alcohol Use, Binge Drinking, and Abuse and Dependence by Adults

	Any alcohol in past 30 days	5 or more drinks in past 30 days	Alcohol abuse or dependence	Illicit drug abuse or dependence
18- to 25-year-olds	60.5	41.2	17.4	8.3
26 and older	53.0	21.1	6.3	1.8

Sources: Office of Applied Studies, Substance Abuse and Mental Health Services Administration. 2005. National household survey on drug use and health. Tables H21 and H38. http://oas.samhsa.gov/nsduh/2k4nsduh/2k4Results/appH.htm#tabh.21 or tabh.38.

by adults is a regulated but legal activity. However, alcohol use by minors is not legal. Second, as will be seen later in this chapter, there is a very clear relationship between underage drinking and the initiation of illicit drug use. Therefore, even if the mandate of ONCDP never changes, there is a logical reason to discuss underage drinking because of the relationship to illicit drug use. Finally, it is important to focus on underage drinking as a significant problem without confounding the issue with the legal use of alcohol by adults.

However, this does not mean that policy changes with regard to alcohol use by adults should be ignored. In Chapter 9, this topic will be discussed.

Why Should the NDCS Focus on Underage Drinking?

Results from the Monitoring the Future Survey show that, in 2005, twice as many 8th–12th graders had used alcohol in the past 30 days compared to the number who had used any illicit drug (see Tables 2.3 and 2.6).[4] That is hardly surprising because alcohol is more available than illicit drugs. However, remember that alcohol is just as illegal for 8th–12th graders as illicit drugs. Of greater concern is the number of young people engaging in binge drinking. The Monitoring the Future Survey collects data on the percentage of young people who consumed five or more drinks in a row in the past 2 weeks. In 2005 the percentages were as follows (the percentage who had used marijuana in the past 30 days is in parentheses)[5]:

8th: 10.5 (6.6)

10th: 21.0 (15.2)

12th: 28.1 (19.8)

Why Doesn't the NDCS Focus on Underage Drinking? | 89

Drinking this amount of alcohol is not experimentation. A young person who has five or more drinks at one time will be intoxicated. When the number of young people who are binge drinking in the last 2 weeks is compared to the number who have used marijuana in the past month, it would be reasonable to expect that the federal government would be just as, if not more, concerned with underage binge drinking than with marijuana use.

According to the National Academy of Sciences, the social cost of underage drinking is estimated to be $53 billion, including $19 billion from traffic accidents and $29 billion from violent crime.[6] Among young people, alcohol is a key factor in the three leading causes of death—accidents, homicides, and suicides.[7] For example, drinking drivers under the age of 21 are involved in fatal crashes at twice the rate of adult drivers.[8] Young people who drink are less likely to wear a seat belt and, in alcohol-related traffic accidents, there were three times more deaths among youth who were not wearing seat belts compared to those who were.[9] Nearly 40 percent of minors who died from drowning, burns, and falls tested positive for alcohol.[10] Alcohol was involved in 36 percent of homicides involving minors and about 10 percent of suicides.[11]

Due to the effect of alcohol on decision making and inhibitions, it is also a factor in risky sexual behavior by minors. Young people are more likely to engage in consensual sexual activity after drinking and to engage in a wider variety of sexual acts than they had planned.[12] They are less likely to use a condom if they have been drinking.[13] In fact, young people who had their first drink before the age of 13 were more than twice as likely to have unprotected sex.

There is also a connection between underage drinking and illicit drug use. The National Household Survey found that 67 percent of young people who were heavy users of alcohol had used illicit drugs in the past month; 44 percent of binge drinkers had done so; and 25 percent of young people who used alcohol but did not binge drink had used illicit drugs in the past month. Only 5.6 percent of young people who did not use alcohol had used illicit drugs.[14] The Center on Addiction and Substance Abuse found that 90 percent of children and adults who use marijuana smoked cigarettes or drank alcohol first. Furthermore, young people who drank alcohol were 50 times more likely to use cocaine than young people who did not drink alcohol.[15]

As with marijuana, it is reasonable to ask whether there is a cause and effect relationship between underage drinking and illicit drug use or between early drinking and risky behaviors such as unprotected sex at a later age. Just as was discussed with the correlation between marijuana and other behaviors, it is possible that young people who start drinking at an early age are more likely to engage in dangerous behaviors simply because of a propensity for rebellious and/or risky activities. However, unlike the situation with marijuana use by young people, there is a clearly established cause and effect relationship between alcohol consumption and immediate outcomes such as deaths and crime. In addition, changes in policies that reduce alcohol availability (e.g., increases in excise taxes, increasing minimum age to drink) have resulted in reduced traffic deaths, crime, sexually transmitted diseases, and tobacco and illicit drug use.[16] Therefore, there are tangible benefits to reducing underage drinking.

In spite of these data on the harm caused by alcohol in comparison to illicit drugs, in 2000, $71.1 million was devoted to preventing underage drinking by the federal government while $1.8 billion was allocated to preventing illicit drug use.[17] In the 2006 budget request, the President recommended cuts in underage drinking prevention initiatives in the Department of Education and the Department of Justice.[18] Even in the research area, there is a great disparity between the federal emphasis on alcohol compared to illicit drugs. The 2006 fiscal year budget request for the National Institute on Drug Abuse (NIDA), the federal agency responsible for research on all aspects of prevention and treatment of illicit drugs, was $1.01 billion.[19] The 2006 fiscal year budget request for the National Institute on Alcohol Abuse and Alcoholism, the comparable agency that coordinates alcohol prevention and treatment research, was $440 million, less than half that of NIDA.[20]

The Value of Underage and Excessive Drinking to the Alcohol Industry

In 2003, the Center on Addiction and Substance Abuse published a white paper on "The Economic Value of Underage Drinking and Adult Excessive Drinking to the Alcohol Industry."[21] Prominent scholars, researchers, and statisticians conducted this analysis. The reason why the alcohol industry must focus on underage drinkers is summarized in the report: "The economic reality of the alcohol industry is that it must maintain or increase consumption if it is to ensure future profits. This means that the industry must continually attract new drinkers as current drinkers quit or die."[22] When the data from Table 5.1 is examined, this argument makes sense. As people get older, there is a dramatic decrease in their heavy use of alcohol. The percentage of binge drinkers falls nearly 50 percent from the 18–25 year group to the 26 and older population. Data from the National Household Survey shows that there is a steady increase in the percentage of people who binge drink and are heavy alcohol users (five or more drinks at one sitting, five or more times a month) from age 12 to 21. Thereafter, the percentages begin to decrease nearly every year as people get older. In fact, there is nearly a 24 percent decrease in the percentage of binge drinkers from age 21 to age 26–29 and a 44 percent decrease in the percentage of heavy alcohol users.[23] Clearly then, the alcohol industry has to focus on underage drinkers to maintain alcohol consumption levels.

This report estimates that underage drinkers are responsible for nearly 20 percent of the alcohol consumed in this country. The heaviest adult drinkers consume another 27 percent and other adult excessive alcohol use accounts for over 19 percent of alcohol consumed. Of the $116.2 billion spent on alcohol, $22.5 is by underage drinkers. According to this report, if underage and excessive adult alcohol use were eliminated, the revenues of the alcohol industry would be cut in half.[24] The underage drinkers of today are the excessive drinkers of the future since young people who start drinking before age 15 are four times more likely to become alcoholic than those who do not drink before age 21 and the incidence of an alcohol problem is greatest for young people who begin drinking between the ages of 11 and 14.[25] The average age of beginning to drink for underage drinkers is 14.[26]

The alcohol industry maintains its underage drinking market by developing products that appeal to young people and through marketing. The current youth-oriented product is "alcopop" beverages which are sweet, fruit-flavored, malt-based drinks. Examples are Smirnoff Ice, Skyy Blue, Henry's Hard Lemonade, Jack Daniel's Hard Cola, and Mike's Hard Cranberry Lemonade. In a survey sponsored by the Alcohol Policies Project in the Center for Science in the Public Interest, a nonprofit health advocacy group, 90 percent of young people said that drinking alcopops would make it more likely that they would drink other alcoholic beverages. Twice as many 14- to 16-year-olds preferred alcopops to beer or mixed drinks and 41 percent of 14- to 18-year-olds had tried these beverages. More than half of the young people reported that the appeal of alcopops was the sweet taste, disguised taste of alcohol, and easy-to-drink character.[27] In 2002, the alcohol industry spent over $1.7 billion on advertising, including over $1 billion on television advertising. The beer industry alone spent $972 million on television ads.[28] In comparison, the ONDCP National Media Campaign spent $185 million in 2002 to convince young people to avoid illicit drugs, about one-tenth of what the alcohol industry spent to convince young people to drink. Of course, the alcohol industry claims that it does not target underage drinkers. However, according to a review of literature conducted by the Center on Alcohol Marketing and Youth at Georgetown University, the number of beer and hard liquor advertising in magazines increases with a magazine's youth readership. Furthermore, 12-year-olds who were more aware of beer advertising held more favorable views on drinking and expressed an intention to drink as adults more often than children who were less aware of these ads. Finally, young people who were exposed to and enjoyed alcohol advertisements were more likely to drink than other youth.[29] The alcohol industry does place "responsibility" advertising on television. However, between 2001 and 2003, there were 761,347 product ads for alcohol on television and 24,161 responsibility ads. Alcohol companies spent 27 times more on product ads than on responsibility ads and 12- to 20-year-olds saw 779 commercials encouraging alcohol use compared to 9 discouraging drinking.[30]

The alcohol industry protects its interests in Congress by contributing money to candidates and parties through political action committees. From 2001 to 2002, beer, wine, and liquor political action committees contributed nearly $3.7 million to federal candidates.[31] One of the largest recipients of these funds, Representative Anne Northup, a Republican from Kentucky, had a leading role in defeating the 1999 amendment authorizing underage drinking prevention ads in the ONDCP Media Campaign.[32] The political action committee for the beer industry, the National Beer Wholesalers Association, is currently the seventh largest donor among all political action committees. It ranks number one in contributions to Republicans.[33]

The alcohol industry has had some success in the past in pressuring federal agencies to minimize underage drinking prevention. In 1995, the National Beer Wholesalers Association successfully lobbied a House subcommittee to eliminate the Center for Substance Abuse Prevention's discretionary budget for grants and initiatives.[34] According to an article written in the Wall Street Journal, a lobbyist for the National Beer Wholesalers Association said

> It drives our wholesalers nuts to know that their tax dollars are being used by groups that are trying to drive them out of business . . . This is our response: We want to cut their funding, stop their lobbying and basically end the use of that structure to bash the beer industry.[35]

You may recall in Chapter 1, I referred to a meeting I attended in Washington, D.C., in which an official of a federal agency warned us about discussing increases in excise taxes as a way to reduce the harm caused by alcohol. That official was from the Center for Substance Abuse Prevention. Although the 1995 budget for the Center for Substance Abuse Prevention was not cut in the final budget negotiations, the agency learned 10 years ago that getting on the wrong side of the alcohol industry means there will be a fight for funding in Congress.

What Should the Federal Government Do to Prevent and Reduce Underage Drinking?

As was stated earlier in the chapter, Congress provided funding for a study by the National Academy of Sciences on underage drinking as a way of postponing action on a bill to fund an underage drinking prevention media campaign that was opposed by the alcohol industry. A report on the results of this study, along with recommendations, was published in 2003.[36] The recommendations were based on a review of the research literature on effective prevention strategies.

Before discussing these recommendations (and noting that Congress has not acted on any of them), the reaction of federal officials and the alcohol industry to the study should be noted. In an editorial in 2003, a journalist connected to a substance abuse prevention research institute wrote:

> the alcohol industry and its supporters in Congress and the administration have conducted a campaign of intimidation against the NAS [National Academy of Sciences] and the committee of experts that wrote the study. NAS officials say they've never seen such intense industry interest in one of their reports. Industry lobbyists are going all-out, and in the forefront of their assault is, as might be expected, the National Beer Wholesalers Association ... While the beer wholesalers and other industry groups publicly supported the study when Congress approved it, they immediately went on the offensive as soon as the research panel was chosen. Rehr [lobbyist for the National Beer Wholesalers Association] and other industry association leaders complained in a letter to NAS administrators last August that the panel was biased, and they named five panel members they insisted were particularly objectionable. This spring the assault intensified. The beer wholesalers began issuing press releases accusing the NAS of misusing taxpayer money by choosing a panel of "controversial individuals" who focused on antiquated or untested solutions in order to "vilify a legal industry," although no panel members had made any public statements about the study, nor had information about the study been released. Next came a letter signed by 138 members of Congress sent to the NAS president, warning him that the $500,000 appropriation was not intended to produce policy changes that would adversely affect the alcohol industry. In February, a Health and Human Services administrator wrote to the study's program officer asking that the alcohol industry be allowed to peer-review the report before it was released. Such a bold request on behalf of an industry with a clear financial interest stunned the research community. Had the program officer allowed this unprecedented intrusion, which she didn't, it would have compromised the scientific integrity of the report and tarnished the entire NAS research progress.[37]

The recommendations from National Academy of Sciences report on underage drinking were as follows[38]:

1. Development of a national adult-oriented media campaign: Since young people frequently obtain alcohol from adults, the purpose of this media campaign would be to encourage adults to take actions to reduce underage drinking and to decrease adult behaviors that facilitate underage drinking (e.g., allowing minors to drink at home).

2. Formation of a partnership to prevent underage drinking: This independent, nonprofit foundation would be funded by the alcohol industry, along with private and public partners, with a mission to reduce and prevent underage drinking.

3. Changing alcohol advertising: The alcohol industry was encouraged to refrain from marketing practices that appeal to underage drinkers and to take precautions to reduce the exposure of young people to alcohol advertising and other marketing activities. It was suggested that an independent external review board be formed to investigate complaints and enforce advertising codes and that existing codes be strengthened against practices which seem to be directed to minors. Congress was asked to fund regular reports on underage exposure to alcohol advertising.

4. Changing the entertainment industry: A rating system and some marketing codes were suggested to reduce underage exposure to entertainment (movies, music, television) with unsuitable alcohol content. Furthermore, the film rating board was encouraged to give mature ratings to movies with unsuitable alcohol content or ones that favorably portray underage drinking. Similarly, it was recommended that television broadcasters and producers take precautions against portraying underage drinking positively. The music industry was asked to avoid glamorizing underage drinking and to develop a rating system similar to that used by other entertainment media. Finally, it was recommended that Congress fund regular reviews of entertainment with large youth audiences to determine the nature and frequency of alcohol use in the content of the entertainment.

5. Limiting the access of underage drinkers to alcohol: There were more recommendations in this section of the report than any in other section. In conjunction with a minimum drinking age of 21, states were encouraged to prohibit adults from supplying alcohol to any children, except their own children in their home. Underage drinking in private establishments should be prohibited. Regular, comprehensive compliance checks of retail alcohol outlets were suggested with an increasing level of sanctions for violations, including license revocation for third

offenses. Federal mandates should be enacted regarding rates of retail compliance with prohibiting sales to minors. Those who sell or serve alcohol should be required to complete a training program as a condition of employment. States were encouraged to enact or strengthen laws that allow negligence law suits against a retailer that sells alcohol to a minor who subsequently injures someone. In addition, states should enact laws to ensure that minors do not gain access to alcohol through Internet sales or home delivery, and enforcement programs should be implemented to deter adults from purchasing alcohol for minors. It was suggested that communities require a system of registering beer kegs that includes the identities of purchasers. All states should have zero tolerance policies of alcohol use by minors who are driving, graduated driver licensing laws, and sobriety checkpoints. Community coalitions, including law enforcement, should work together on policies to identify and end underage drinking parties. Finally, there were recommendations regarding the prevention and detection of false identification documents and on penalties for alcohol infractions by minors.

6. Youth-oriented initiatives: Interestingly, the report did not recommend a youth-oriented media campaign because of a lack of evidence regarding the effectiveness of this approach. It was suggested that research be conducted to determine if effective media campaigns can be developed. Only evidence-based underage drinking prevention programs should be funded by federal agencies. There was particular attention to interventions at colleges and universities, including screening to detect problem drinkers and brief interventions with those who are identified, policy enforcement, and strategies to limit access to alcohol. It was recommended that federal agencies expand referral, diagnosis, and treatment services for minors with alcohol problems.

7. Community interventions: The recommendations in this area focused on the development of community coalitions whose primary mission would be to prevent and reduce underage drinking. The report noted that the federal government provides funding for community coalitions that target illicit drug use and suggested a similar funding stream for underage drinking.

8. Government assistance and coordination: The report recommended that the federal government establish an interagency coordinating committee on prevention of underage drinking, establish a national training and research center on underage drinking, issue an annual report on the

subject, and increase national survey data on drinking patterns of youth. In addition, each state should establish a lead agency to coordinate activities on the prevention and reduction of underage drinking.

9. Alcohol excise taxes: The National Academy of Sciences report documented three important points with regard to excise taxes. First, alcoholic beverages, particularly beer, are far cheaper today (after adjusting for inflation) than in the 1960s and 1970s. Second, increasing excise taxes on alcohol has been shown to decrease consumption by minors. Third, research has shown that increasing excise taxes on alcohol decreases the harm caused by underage drinking, including driving fatalities, crime, and sexually transmitted disease. Needless to say, the report recommended an increase in excise taxes on alcohol, with future increases tied to the consumer price index.

10. Research and evaluation: The report recommended rigorous evaluation of all interventions for the prevention and reduction of underage drinking and funding for the development and evaluation of new interventions.

It is not difficult to understand the reasons why the alcohol industry was concerned with the National Academy of Sciences report. If the recommendations were adopted, they would have a detrimental impact on the profits of alcohol companies. Representatives of the committee who conducted the National Academy of Sciences study did testify before the Senate Subcommittee on Substance Abuse and Mental Health Services, Committee on Health, Education, Labor and Pensions, on September 30, 2003. However, the power of the alcohol industry should not be doubted. As the number one political action committee in contributions to the Republican Party, which controlled both houses of Congress, the Beer Wholesalers Association was successful in blocking the implementation of any of the recommendations.

Conclusions

The lack of emphasis on underage drinking in the NDCS is illogical for two reasons. First, the harm from underage drinking is immense, particularly in comparison to illicit drug use. Second, the relationship between underage drinking and illicit drug use is very strong. ONDCP justifies its focus on marijuana based on the inherent dangers of this drug and the relationship between marijuana and other illicit drug use. If this same logic were applied to underage drinking, the NDCS should have a major emphasis on the prevention and reduction of underage drinking.

The reasons why the ONDCP mandate has not been changed by Congress to focus on underage drinking are simple to discern. The alcohol industry makes a great deal of money on underage drinking and excessive drinking by adults who started as underage drinkers. This industry contributes a large amount of money to policy makers to protect its financial interests. Therefore, just as occurs in many other areas, public policy regarding underage drinking is not based on what is logical, but is based on which lobbying group has the most influence. The alcohol industry wins.

In the next chapter, the impact of public policy regarding underage drinking on substance abuse prevention will be discussed. Prior to this analysis, there is an undeniable reality that adults must understand. The prevention of illicit drug use by young people is interwoven with the prevention of underage drinking. Policies to prevent underage drinking will inconvenience adults (e.g., increases in alcohol excise taxes). Thus, if adults resist changes in public policies regarding alcohol that are inconvenient, there is very little chance that illicit drug use by young people will change.

Six

Does Prevention Work?

Introduction

The rationale for substance abuse prevention from a federal perspective is described in the 2002 NDCS:

> Common sense tells us that preventing young people from experimenting with drugs in the first place is preferable to later—and more costly—treatment, rehabilitation, and possible incarceration. Preventing drug use before it starts spares families the anguish of watching a relative slip into the grasp of addiction and protects society from many risks, such as those created by workers whose mental faculties are dulled by chemicals. Prevention is also the most cost-effective approach to the drug problem, sparing society the burden of treatment, rehabilitation, lost productivity, and other social pathologies—costs estimated at $160 billion per year.[1]

In other words, if prevention efforts were effective, there should be a reduction in the personal, social, familial, societal, and economic harm of drug abuse and addiction. That makes sense. However, as was seen in Chapter 2, there is no evidence that there has been a reduction in the consequences of drug abuse and addiction (e.g., emergency room visits, crime) in the past 10 years. Therefore, it is certainly reasonable to question whether the prevention activities and strategies supported by ONDCP over the last decade have been effective.

In this chapter, there will be an examination of the current prevention activities supported through the NDCS, analysis of the reasons why these activities have not produced the desired effects, and suggestions for alternatives that may make prevention more effective. However, before there can be an understanding of the reasons why the prevention strategies of the NDCS have not worked, aspects of substance abuse prevention must be understood.

What Exactly Is Substance Abuse Prevention?

When most people think about substance abuse prevention, they think of Nancy Reagan's "Just Say No," or some type of school-based program like the Drug Abuse Resistance Education (DARE) program, in which police officers provide instruction to 5th-grade students on drugs and guide activities to build social skills and self-esteem. However, neither of these efforts would be considered to be effective substance abuse prevention by professionals in the field. Effective substance abuse prevention activities should have research evidence that supports their success (neither "Just Say No" nor DARE fit this criterion) and should be comprehensive, involving many segments of a community and a variety of activities.[2]

An effective, comprehensive prevention program includes activities that can be categorized into six strategies[3]:

1. *Information dissemination* is communication regarding the facts about drugs, consequences of drug abuse, resources, and services. A lecture about the dangers of illicit drugs or brochures on this topic would be examples of information dissemination.

2. *Prevention education* involves interactive activities regarding social and life skills, such as decision making, making friends, and refusal skills (i.e., how to say "no" and keep your friends).

3. *Alternative activities*, such as participation in alcohol and drug-free events or healthy pursuits that are incompatible with drug use, is another strategy. Midnight basketball, in which organized games are held in urban area gyms late at night, is a well-known example of an alternative activity.

4. *Community-based processes* involve activities such as developing community coalitions, interagency collaborations, and networking. For example, a community may decide to organize a coalition involving public schools, the faith community, service groups, social service agencies, law enforcement, and the business community to plan and implement substance abuse prevention initiatives.

5. *Environmental approaches* are the laws, policies, and regulations involving tobacco, alcohol, and other drugs. Increasing the excise tax on alcohol or

restricting retail outlets licensed to sell alcohol are examples of environ- mental prevention approaches.

6. *Problem identification and referral* means identifying individuals who have used substances inappropriately or illegally and determining the best course of action. For example, a student drug testing program may identify students who have used illicit drugs. Following identification, the student would be referred for an assessment to determine if he or she needed treatment for drug abuse or addiction.

In addition to the different types of strategies, substance abuse prevention activities can have different target groups, described as universal, selective, or indi- cated populations. Universal prevention strategies are implemented for groups as a whole. No person is chosen to participate because of an increased risk for substance abuse. A prevention program taught to all 6th graders at a school and antidrug messages on television are examples of programs targeted to universal populations. The goal is to provide all the members of the group with the knowledge and/or skills to prevent substance abuse. Selective prevention strategies target a subset of a group that is at risk for substance use because of some characteristic they share. For example, children whose parents are alcoholics or drug addicts are at higher risk for substance abuse than children whose parents are moderate users of alcohol. A support group for these children would be an example of a selective prevention strategy. An individual member of this "at risk" subgroup may not be exhibiting any behavior that indicates he or she is on the way to abusing substances. The individual is chosen to participate in the prevention strategy only because he or she possesses a characteristic that increases the probability of later substance abuse. An indicated prevention strategy is directed toward individuals who demonstrate a behavior or characteristic that is predictive of later substance abuse. Elementary school students who are caught smoking would be an example. A prevention strategy for these children might involve an education/counseling group.

As can be seen, substance abuse prevention involves many different types of activities and these activities can have a variety of target audiences, depending on the purpose of the activity. As we review what is currently being supported in the prevention area through the NDCS, it is important to remember that the most effective prevention programs are comprehensive, incorporating activities from multiple strategies.[4]

A Theoretical Model of Prevention

The most widely accepted theoretical conceptualization for substance abuse prevention is called the risk and protective factors theory, conceived by David

Hawkins and Richard Catalano at the University of Washington.[5] This model was developed from a review of 30 years of research on youth substance abuse and delinquency and is used by the Center for Substance Abuse Prevention, the major federal agency involved with drug prevention, in the development of initiatives.[6] Therefore, it is important to understand this theory.

The risk and protective factors theory is analogous to the medical model of assessing the risk for heart disease. An individual has certain risk factors for heart disease such as a family history of heart disease, smoking, and obesity. While people can't change their genes, they can reduce their risk of heart disease by quitting smoking and losing weight. Similarly, there are protective factors, such as exercise and taking vitamins, which can decrease the probability of heart disease, even for people with a family history of this condition. So, a young person's risk for later substance abuse can be determined by the number of risk factors that are present in his or her life. Theoretically, the risk could be reduced by minimizing or eliminating these risk factors. Furthermore, a young person's risk for later substance abuse can be mitigated by the enhancement of the identified protective factors.

The risk factors have been categorized as follows: community risk factors, family risk factors, school risk factors, and individual/peer risk factors. The protective factors are categorized as individual characteristics, bonding, and healthy beliefs and clear standards. It should be noted that most of the risk factors have also been shown to be risk factors for other youth problems, such as delinquency, teen pregnancy, school dropout, and youth violence.[7]

The following is a description of the risk and protective factors.[8]

Community Risk Factors

Availability of drugs—The more available drugs are in the community, the higher the risk that young people will abuse drugs in the community. Perceived availability of drugs is also associated with risk. In schools where children just think that drugs are more available, a higher rate of drug use occurs.

Community laws and norms favorable toward drug use—Community norms are communicated through laws and written policies, informal social practices, and the expectations parents and other members of the community have of young people. An example of a community law is the taxation of alcoholic beverages. Conflicting messages from parents and social institutions can result in ambiguity for young people. For example, acceptance of alcohol at community social events is in conflict with "just say no" messages from parents and schools.

Transitions and mobility—Normal school transitions, such as the move from elementary to middle school, as well as nonscheduled transitions, are predictive of increases in drug use, school misbehavior, and delinquency. An increased risk of drug use and crime is associated with high rates of mobility in a community.

Low neighborhood attachment and community disorganization—In communities and neighborhoods where residents have little attachment to their area, there are higher rates of drug problems, juvenile delinquency, and violence. The degree of community attachment is related to the homogeneity of the neighborhood, the degree to which residents believe they can control their destinies, and the extent to which merchants, teachers, police, and social service workers live in the community. Attachment to the community is also related to the degree of voter turnout and parental involvement in schools.

Extreme economic deprivation—Children who live in deteriorating, crime-ridden neighborhoods characterized by extreme poverty and who have behavior and adjustment problems early in life are more likely to have problems with drugs.

Family Risk Factors

Family history of the problem behavior—If children are raised in a family with a history of alcohol or other drug addiction, the children have an increased risk for later substance abuse.

Family management problems—Poor family management practices include lack of clear expectations for behavior, failure to monitor children (e.g., knowing where they are and who they are with), and excessively severe or inconsistent punishment.

Family conflict—Regardless of family constellation, persistent, serious conflict between primary caregivers or between caregivers and children increases the risk for substance abuse by children in the family.

Parental attitudes and involvement in drug use, crime, and violence—In families where parents involve children in their own alcohol or other drug behavior (e.g., asking the child to light the parent's cigarette or get the parent a beer), there is an increased risk of later drug abuse by the children. Parental approval of moderate drinking by minors, even under parental supervision, is associated with an increased risk of the use of marijuana by the children.

School Risk Factors

Early and persistent antisocial behavior—Male children who are aggressive in primary grades (K-3) are at greater risk for substance abuse. When aggressive behavior is combined with isolation, hyperactivity, or attention deficit disorder, the risk is even greater for adolescent substance abuse. This risk factor includes persistent problem behaviors in early adolescence, such as skipping school and fighting.

Academic failure beginning in elementary school—This risk factor involves the experience of academic failure, regardless of the cause of the failure. Therefore, it does not matter if the academic failure is the result of poor teaching, cultural or language issues, or a disability. The risk for later substance abuse is increased for any cause of academic failure.

Lack of commitment to school—Low commitment to school involves lack of engagement in the academic and extracurricular activities at school. The student does not perceive the value of education.

Individual/Peer Risk Factors

Alienation/rebelliousness—Young people who feel they are not part of society, who act as if they were not bound by rules, who do not believe in trying to be successful or responsible, or who take an active rebellious stance toward society are at high risk for drug abuse.

Friends who engage in problem behavior—Associating with peers who use drugs is one of the most consistent predictors of later substance abuse, even among children with a low number of other risk factors. However, young people with a low number of other risk factors are less likely to associate with peers who use drugs.

Favorable attitudes toward the problem behavior—During elementary school, children generally express antidrug, anticrime, and prosocial attitudes. However, in middle school, their attitudes often shift toward greater acceptance of problem behaviors, presumably due to the fact that they increasingly know others who engage in these behaviors. An accepting attitude toward drug use is a predictor of later substance abuse problems.

Early initiation of the problem behavior—The earlier a child begins to use tobacco, alcohol, or other drugs, the greater the risk of later substance abuse problems.

Constitutional factors—There is evidence that personality characteristics such as sensation-seeking, poor impulse control, and low avoidance of harm are biologically based. These characteristics are associated with an increased risk of later substance abuse. In addition, it is likely that there is a genetic component to addiction.

Protective Factors

Individual characteristics—The four protective characteristics include gender (females have greater protection), a resilient temperament, a positive social orientation, and high intelligence. However, high intelligence alone does not protect a person from alcoholism or drug addiction, as many bright alcoholics and addicts can attest.

Bonding—Children who are attached to positive families, friends, schools, and communities, and who are committed to achieving the goals valued by these groups are less likely to develop problems in adolescence. For effective bonding to occur, the child must have meaningful opportunities to contribute to their community, school, family, and peer group; the skills to take advantage of the opportunities; and recognition for efforts to contribute.

Healthy beliefs and clear standards—The people to whom children are bonded need to have clear, positive standards for behavior. The content of these standards is what protects young people. When parents, teachers, and communities set clear standards for children's behavior, when the standards are widely and consistently supported, and when the consequences for not following the standards are consistent, the young people are more likely to follow the standards.

Although the information in this section is condensed, it provides the basic framework for the implementation of substance abuse prevention in communities. Theoretically, a community coalition would conduct an assessment to determine the most pressing risk factors to target and the extent to which protective factors can be enhanced. Prevention programs and activities from each of the six strategies would be chosen to reduce the targeted risk factors and to enhance the protective factors. The prevention programs and activities would be directed to universal, selective, or indicated populations, depending on the needs in the community. Hopefully, the prevention programs and activities that are chosen would be those that research has shown to be the most effective.[9]

The Prevention Activities in the NDCS

Five federal agencies are involved with the implementation of the vast majority of prevention initiatives in the NDCS. The activities in each of these agencies will be described, as well as the agency budgets from fiscal year 2004 to fiscal year 2006.[10] There is also a mechanism to determine the effectiveness of most of these programs. Since 2002, the federal government has used something called the Program Assessment Rating Tool (PART) to evaluate a program's purpose, planning, management, and results. A program can receive a score from 0 to 100 on each of the four dimensions. However, not all of these programs have been evaluated with PART. In addition, the Government Performance and Results Act (GPRA) requires agencies to set targets and to evaluate their efforts in relation to these targets.

National Institute on Drug Abuse (NIDA)[11]

NIDA, a part of the Department of Health and Human Services, provides funding for prevention and treatment research. The prevention research budget for 2006 was $409.0 million, an increase of about $2 million over 2005 and $6.3 million more than in 2004. In 2005, NIDA supported research on how to prevent the escalation from early drug use to regular use, abuse, and addiction, and the role of primary healthcare professionals in drug abuse prevention. In 2006, NIDA will fund research on "Understanding the neurobiological consequences of environmental stressors during childhood and adolescence as it pertains to drug use and addiction . . ." because this research ". . . is essential to drug abuse prevention efforts."[12] For example, this type of research might investigate chemical changes in the brains of youth that occur in response to a stressful situation (e.g., abuse) and the relationship between these chemical changes and the chemical changes that result from drug craving. Of course, any research that is looking at chemical changes in the brain must use animal subjects rather than human subjects, so "youth" would probably involve adolescent rats and "abuse" might be induced by electric shocks. It remains to be seen whether or not this type of research is "essential to drug abuse prevention efforts." However, regardless of the outcomes, this type of research is years away from having an impact on substance abuse prevention.

There has not been a PART review of NIDA up to now. The GPRA targets set by NIDA all involve treatment. NIDA did not establish any GPRA targets for prevention research.

Office of Justice Programs[13]

The Office of Justice Programs in the Department of Justice received $31.7 million for prevention in 2004, $31.0 in 2005, and $29.5 in 2006. The President's budget request for 2006 was $12.5 million. The decrease was due to the elimination of the Underage Drinking Prevention Program, a grant program for states to support efforts to prohibit the sale of alcoholic beverages to minors and the purchase and consumption of alcoholic beverages by minors. However, Congress maintained the funding of this program. The remainder of the prevention money is allocated to a program called "Weed and Seed," which involves a combination of law enforcement and community-based services in high-crime neighborhoods. The only PART assessment for the Office of Justice Programs involves treatment and will be discussed in the following chapter.

U.S. Department of Education[14]

The U.S. Department of Education has had two substance abuse prevention programs, the Safe and Drug-Free Schools and Communities (SDFSC) State Grants and the SDFSC National Programs. In 2004 and 2005, the SDFSC State Grants received $440.9 million and $437.4 million respectively. These funds are given to governors (20 percent) and State Educational Agencies (80 percent). The State Educational Agencies are required to distribute 93 percent of the funds to Local Education Agencies (i.e., school districts) "... for a wide variety of activities to prevent or reduce violence and delinquency and the use, possession, and distribution of illegal drugs, and thereby foster a safe and drug-free learning environment that supports academic achievement."[15] The 2006 budget recommended that this program be eliminated because the 2004 PART review gave the program an "ineffective" rating "... due to the program's inability to demonstrate effectiveness and the fact that grant funds are spread too thinly to support quality interventions."[16] The program's purpose received a score of 60, planning 57, management 38, and results 0. As was previously stated, these scores are out of a possible score of 100. This program has been in the Department of Education's budget during the entire 10-year period discussed in this book. Congress did not eliminate this program in the 2006 budget but did reduce funding by about $90 million.

The SDFSC National Programs provide funding for various grants and national initiatives. This program received over $153 million in 2004 and 2005 and nearly $233 million was requested for 2006. The President requested an additional $87.5 million from the 2005 budget to "... implement research-based drug prevention grants for local educational agencies."[17] However, Congress reduced the 2005 budget by about $9 million. In addition, $32.7 million was recommended to be cut from the Alcohol Abuse Reduction Program, grants to local school districts to implement evidenced-based programs to reduce underage drinking. No reason for this cut is provided in the ONDCP budget request. Again, Congress did not follow the President's recommendation. Finally, $25.4 million, an increase of $15.4 million over the 2005 budget, was requested to triple the number of grants for school-based drug testing. Congress authorized $10.4 million for this program. It should be noted that a 2003 review of drug testing practices in schools found that "Drug testing was not associated with students' reported illicit drug use, or with rate of use among experienced marijuana users. Drug testing of athletes was not associated with illicit drug use among male high school athletes."[18] This literature review and analysis was conducted by the researchers who are involved with the Monitoring the Future survey, so it would be difficult to argue that they were biased against an ONDCP program.

There were no PART evaluations for the SDFSC National Programs. However, a target was set of a 5 percent annual reduction in drug use in the target population of students among school drug testing grantees.

Substance Abuse and Mental Health Services Administration (SAMHSA)[19, 20]

SAMHSA is in Health and Human Services and is made up of three centers, including the Center for Substance Abuse Prevention (CSAP) that, obviously, implements the prevention activities for SAMHSA. The 2006 budget was $563.0 million which was about $9.5 million less than 2004 and 2005. Of this amount, $351.7 million was provided for the Block Grant, slightly less than the last 2 years. These are funds that are distributed to states for prevention and treatment services. The money is given to the Single State Authority in each state responsible for substance abuse prevention and treatment and distributed to local programs in each state depending on its own structure and system. The $351.7 million represents a 20 percent set aside of the Block Grant which must, by law, be used for prevention. According to the ONDCP budget document

> CSAP requires under regulation that the States use their Block Grant funds to support a range of prevention services and activities in six key areas to ensure that each State offers a comprehensive system for preventing substance abuse. The six areas are information dissemination, community-based process, environmental strategies, alternative activities, education, and problem identification and referral. The Block Grant funds are the foundation of most States' prevention systems, driving their prevention planning processes and setting standards and priorities for their overall prevention systems.[21]

The 2003 PART evaluation rated the Block Grant as "ineffective." Purpose received a score of 80, planning 50, management 89, and results 8. According to the PART evaluation, "Without uniformly-defined and collected outcome information from each state, the program (including prevention and treatment) could not demonstrate its effectiveness."[22] However, according to ONDCP "SAMHSA has made progress in working with the states to identify a set of 'national outcomes' that will be monitored across all SAMHSA programs."[23] Parenthetically, I have been personally involved in many of these discussions about outcomes, data management, and reporting and it has been going on for about 4 years. It should also be noted that the Block Grant has been funded for the entire 10-year period discussed in this book (and more) without any outcome measures to determine effectiveness.

The other CSAP funding category is called Programs of Regional and National Significance. The 2006 budget was $192.9 million, about $6 million less than the previous 2 years. Much of this money will be devoted to the Strategic Prevention Framework State Incentive Grants program. This will provide about $2.35 million annually to 19 states continuing for a third year, 5 states for a second year, and 12–15 new awards. According to ONDCP

The Strategic Prevention Framework incorporates a five step community development model: 1) organize the community to profile needs, including community readiness; 2) mobilize the community and build the capacity to address needs and plan for sustainability; 3) develop the prevention action (evidence-based activities, programs, strategies, and policies); 4) implement the prevention plan; and 5) conduct ongoing evaluation for quality improvements and outcomes. The Strategic Prevention Framework is based upon the risk and protective factor approach to prevention.[24]

The Strategic Prevention Framework was not evaluated through PART. It should be noted that this program replaced an earlier State Incentive Grant program described in Chapter 2. This program provided approximately $9 million over 3 years to nearly every state to assist community-based programs in the implementation of evidence-based prevention programs. According to ONDCP, "The program (State Incentive Grant) consistently exceeded the target of increasing the number of evidence-based programs implemented. However, data collection efforts were less successful with respect to other outcomes."[25] In other words, the community-based organizations implemented evidence-based programs, but it is unclear if this did any good. That program cost about $350 million.

The second largest program in the Programs of Regional and National Significance is the Substance Abuse Prevention and HIV Prevention in Minority Communities Services Grant. In 2006, $39.4 million was requested to support 139 grants. According to ONDCP, "This program is designed to increase prevention services capacity in minority communities, which are disproportionately impacted by HIV disease."[26] This program, ". . . is undergoing major review as well, with changes expected as the request for applications is issued for FY 2005. The current program has experienced difficulty collecting data for performance measurement, and as the program is reassessed, data and performance measurement issues will be resolved."[27]

The only other program with specific references to performance is the Centers for the Application of Prevention Technologies, with a budget request in 2006 of $11.7 million, nearly the same amount allocated in 2004 and 2005.[28] These five regional centers provide training and technical assistance for states, grant recipients, and community-based organizations and have been in existence since 1997. According to ONDCP, "The Centers for the Application of Prevention Technologies exceeded the 2004 target for increasing the number of person [*sic*] provided technical assistance services by employing more efficient, technologically sophisticated technical assistance delivery methods."[29]

The PART evaluation for the Programs of Regional and National Significance rated this section "moderately effective":

> The program makes a unique contribution by focusing on regional, emerging problems. The program is developing two primary long-term outcome measures, which are already being used at the national level in the ONDCP National Drug Control Strategy and in Healthy People 2010 and directly measure the program's purpose to reduce and prevent substance abuse.[30]

The purpose of Programs of Regional and National Significance received a score of 100, planning 88, management 90, and results 47.

Office of National Drug Control Policy[31]

There are two major prevention programs funded through ONDCP, the Media Campaign and the Drug-Free Communities Support Program. The Media Campaign received $144.1 million in 2004, $119.0 in 2005, and $120 million was requested for the 2006 budget. However, Congress only allocated $99 million. The program is described by ONDCP as follows:

> The Media Campaign is an integrated effort that combines TV, radio, print, and interactive media with public communications outreach to youth and parents. Anti-drug messages conveyed in national advertising are supported by web sites, media events, outreach to the entertainment industry, and the formation of strategic partnerships with public health organizations, NGOs, and other government and private sector entities that enable the anti-drug messages to be amplified in ways that personally resonate with audiences. In particular, the Media Campaign focuses the majority of its efforts on educating 14- to 16-year-olds and their parents on the negative consequences of using marijuana . . .[32]

In Chapter 2, it was noted that the Media Campaign began in 1997 as part of the Clinton administration's Youth Substance Abuse Prevention Initiative. That year, $175 million was allocated to the Media Campaign. From 1997 to 2006, over $1.5 billion will have been spent on the Media Campaign. In describing the performance of the Media Campaign, ONDCP reported:

> The FY2005 PART review found that the Media Campaign program had made improvements in planning and management, including the establishment of reasonable and measurable performance goals. However, the results of the independent evaluation (managed by NIDA) detected no connection between the program advertisements and youth attitudes and behavior toward drug use. Other evidence, such as findings from MTF, NSDUH, and PATS, suggest there maybe [sic] a positive effect on youth attitudes and behavior.[33]

Interestingly, the PART assessment for the Media Campaign was not printed in the ONDCP budget document, in contrast to the PART assessments for other federal agencies. However, PART assessments are public documents and can be accessed through the Office of Management and Budget Web site.[34] The Media Campaign was rated "Results Not Demonstrated." The scores were as follows: purpose 100, planning 67, management 70, results 6.

The Drug-Free Communities Support Program:

> ... supports the development and expansion of community anti-drug coalitions throughout the United States. Initially created as a five-year program (FY 1998 through FY 2002) authorized by the Drug-Free Communities Act of 1997, the program was re-authorized by Congress for an additional five-year period that will extend the program through FY 2007. The program provides up to $100,000 per year in grant funding to local community, anti-drug coalition, which must be matched by local communities ... Community coalitions typically strive to increase community involvement and effectiveness in carrying out a wide array of drug prevention strategies, initiatives, and activities ...[35]

Since 1997, there has been a gradual increase in funding for the Drug-Free Communities Support program as more and more coalitions have been awarded grants. In 2004, $69.6 million was allocated for this program, $79.4 million in 2005, and $79.2 million in 2006. The 2005 PART assessment was "adequate" with scores of 100 for purpose, 50 in planning, 80 for management, and 42 for results. The comments were, "Program management is strong. Baselines and targets are needed. Performance information should be made public."[36]

In summary, the five major federal agencies involved with substance abuse prevention (National Institute on Drug Abuse, Office of Justice Programs, Department of Education, Substance Abuse and Mental Health Services Administration, Office of National Drug Control Policy) have spent or are planning to spend nearly $5 billion on prevention research and activities from 2004 through 2006. In the research area, there has not been a PART review and none of the targets of the funding agency (National Institute on Drug Abuse) involve prevention. In the Office of Justice Programs, grants to states to combat underage drinking were proposed for elimination without explanation. The major program funded by the U.S. Department of Education for more than 10 years has been judged ineffective and was recommended to be eliminated. A program to reduce underage drinking was slated to be cut by the administration for no apparent reason and a program on drug testing in schools was recommended for increased funding, in spite of research evidence that such programs are not successful in reducing drug use. The largest source of prevention funding, the Block Grant funded by the Center for Substance Abuse Prevention in the Substance Abuse and Mental Health Administration, has been evaluated as ineffective because of an inability, despite years of effort, to design and implement a system to collect outcome data. This same agency spent hundreds of millions of dollars in giving states grants to implement evidence-based prevention programs in their communities and is now spending hundreds of millions of dollars more on an entirely new program to give money to these same states for nearly the same purpose after the first program could not demonstrate effectiveness. ONDCP has spent $1.5 billion on a national media campaign that another federal agency has evaluated and found to be ineffective. A 10-year program to support community coalitions, funded by specific legislation, was only evaluated as adequate and was criticized for not making performance information available to the public.

What Is the Problem?

Administrative and Implementation Issues

At the beginning of this chapter, it was noted that there is a lack of evidence that prevention has successfully reduced the harms and consequences of substance abuse. However, the substance abuse prevention field has a research-based theoretical model of risk and protective factors to guide it, a conceptualization of strategies for program implementation, and research on what types of activities work and don't work. In addition, the federal government has spent a considerable amount of money on prevention. Why isn't this whole effort more successful?

At a simple level, government ineptitude, bureaucratic intransigence, and politics might be suspected. Based on my personal experiences with three of the five agencies involved with prevention (I have had very little contact with the National Institute on Drug Abuse or the Office of Justice Programs), these factors certainly exist. The inability of the Center for Substance Abuse Prevention to develop and implement an efficient data management system to measure outcomes of substance abuse prevention at the state and community levels has been due to poor leadership, bureaucratic infighting, and personnel issues. For example, several years ago, this agency decided to develop a Web-based system to assist states and communities with determining the most appropriate prevention strategies to implement and a process to measure the outcomes of these strategies. This system was called the "Decision Support System." As part of one of the projects in the center I directed, my staff and I, as well as other staff members from similar projects, were asked to review the concept and various drafts of the Web site. We consistently told the Center for Substance Abuse Prevention staff that the concept was too complex, the Web site unwieldy to navigate, and that states and community-based prevention providers would not use it. In spite of this feedback, the project went forward. Several federal bureaucrats at the Center for Substance Abuse Prevention were invested in the project and not willing to listen to criticism. Over $1 million was spent for the development of the Web site. Today, it doesn't exist. As predicted, it was too difficult to use. Eventually, the Center for Substance Abuse Prevention terminated the Web site, wasting many hours and many taxpayer dollars. I was present at the first unveiling of commercials for the National Media Campaign in 1997. Those of us who saw the commercials (and who weren't federal employees) were mostly amused by the efforts and appalled by the amount of money being spent. Given our knowledge of prevention and adolescent development, there was no doubt that these messages would be ineffective. Now $1.5 billion later, the PART assessment validates this opinion. The student drug testing initiative is being driven by a political agenda to be "tough on drugs." As was stated, the research evidence does not support student drug testing as an effective means to reduce drug use. Also, logic would lead one to question student drug testing. If a group of high school students, athletes for example, know that there will be random drug testing but no testing for alcohol, they will probably drink instead of smoking marijuana. In that case, nothing has been accomplished by drug testing, even if marijuana smoking is reduced among the student athletes.

However, federal incompetence, bureaucracy, and politics cannot totally explain the lack of impact of substance abuse prevention. Even if programs have not been systematically gathering outcome data, evidence-based prevention programs and strategies have been implemented in communities across the country through initiatives such as the State Incentive Grant Program and Drug-Free Communities Support Program. Therefore, some impact on the harm and consequences of drug abuse would be expected if these programs were working effectively, in spite of the federal government's problems in administering these programs. However, as has been seen, the data on the consequences of drug abuse and of the harm caused by drug abuse has not improved over the 10-year period of time that has been examined.

Perhaps there are issues at the community level in the implementation of evidence-based prevention programs and strategies. Again, I have some personal experience that leads me to believe that this is part of the problem. One of the missions of the Center for the Application of Prevention Technologies (a program in the center I directed funded by the Center for Substance Abuse Prevention) is to help communities implement evidence-based programs and strategies. In many cases, because of state or grant requirements, community-based organizations must choose an evidence-based program from a registry administered by the Substance Abuse and Mental Health Services Administration called the "National Registry of Evidence-based Programs and Practices."[37] A program gets on this registry after documenting that it has been proven to be effective through a rigorous evaluation. Most of the programs on the registry have been started with grant funds, so they generally have had money to hire well-trained staff, to provide the needed materials and supplies, and to have the necessary support staff to implement the program. However, the community-based organizations that are adopting these evidence-based programs frequently do not have the same level of resources. So, they often want to "adapt" the program by shortening it, using volunteers or less-qualified staff, or otherwise cutting corners. Sometimes the evidence-based program was developed in a community that is very different demographically than the community that wants to adopt it. Therefore, we would find that community-based organizations often implemented a version of an evidence-based program but not the identical program. So, part of the problem with demonstrating the impact of substance abuse prevention may be that evidence-based programs are not really being implemented with fidelity.

While the issues discussed thus far probably contribute to the fact that prevention has not reduced the harm caused by drug abuse, these issues do not fully explain the situation. At the state and community levels, well-intentioned and hardworking people are often able to overcome federal ineptitude. Furthermore, I have personally seen many state prevention systems and community-based organizations doing an exemplary job of using a risk and protective framework to design and implement evidence-based prevention programs. There must be other factors that explain the failure of substance abuse prevention.

Utility of the Risk and Protective Factor Theory

As was previously stated, the risk and protective factor theory is the most widely used conceptualization to guide substance abuse prevention. However, the basic premise of the theory is that the risk factors are *predictive* of later substance abuse. In other words, the more risk factors a young person has, the greater the likelihood of that young person developing an alcohol or drug problem later in life. That does not mean that the risk factors *cause* substance abuse problems. Remember the statistics cliché, "Correlation does not imply causation?" The risk factors are correlated with later substance abuse. So, if there is not a causal relationship between risk factors and later substance abuse problems, prevention efforts that are directed at reducing risk factors may not have any impact on alcohol and drug abuse. Whether or not a cause and effect relationship exists between the risk factors and substance abuse is unknown, mainly because there is such a long time period between the risk factor and the evidence of a substance abuse problem. For example, a school risk factor is academic failure that begins in elementary school. However, an adolescent substance abuse problem is usually exhibited in high school. It would be very difficult to establish a cause and effect relationship between the academic failure that occurred at the age of 8 and a drug problem that was diagnosed at age 16.

More importantly perhaps, are the risk factors themselves and what they represent. Of the 17 risk factors, 14 are related to socioeconomic status, community dysfunction, and family issues: transitions and mobility, low neighborhood attachment and community disorganization, extreme economic deprivation, family history of the problem behavior, family management problems, family conflict, parental attitudes and involvement in drug use, early and persistent antisocial behavior, academic failure beginning in elementary school, lack of commitment to school, alienation/rebelliousness, friends who engage in the problem behavior, favorable attitudes toward the problem behavior, and early initiation of the problem behavior. These seem like problems in our society related to poverty and the deterioration of family structures. It may be reasonable to suspect that these risk factors are related in a causal fashion to later substance abuse problems, even if this relationship is difficult to prove scientifically. However, even if such a causal relationship exists, our society has not been very successful in reducing these risk factors. Furthermore, it isn't logical to think that a young person with several of these risk factors is going to be convinced to stay away from drugs by the federal programs discussed here. For example, is it likely that a child who lives in poverty in a deteriorating, violent community with a parent who uses drugs is going to develop a positive attitude toward drug use through seeing Media Campaign commercials on television? It is no surprise that these risk factors are also predictive of delinquency, violence, and teen pregnancy. They are illustrative of persistent, entrenched problems that have plagued a large segment of American society for many years. It is not realistic to expect substance abuse prevention efforts alone to impact these risk factors.

The Impact of Alcohol Marketing

As was stated in the previous chapter, in 2002, ONDCP spent $180 million on the media campaign to convince young people not to use drugs. In 2002, the alcohol industry spent $1.7 billion on advertising or nearly 10 times what ONDCP spent.[38] In 2006, the media campaign is allocated $99 million. It is not likely that the alcohol industry is spending less than they did in 2002.

As was discussed in Chapter 5, alcohol is a problem in and of itself and as a predictor of illicit drug use. Also, the alcohol industry has a financial interest in underage drinking and targets marketing efforts to minors. If it is possible that substance abuse prevention efforts can have any impact on the development of alcohol and drug abuse problems, this impact is subverted by the marketing of alcohol to underage drinkers. It is like there are two opposing forces, one force is trying to influence young people not to use illicit drugs while the other force is encouraging young people to use alcohol. Unfortunately, the "use alcohol force" is far better financed and much more creative in their advertising than the "don't use illicit drugs force." Furthermore, in the extremely unlikely event that a young person who uses alcohol is convinced by prevention efforts to stay away from illicit drugs, is there a tremendous benefit to the individual or to the society? If that young person has the propensity to develop an addiction problem, he or she may become addicted to alcohol which causes as many or more problems than addiction to illicit drugs. Furthermore, alcohol is a major factor in the harm caused to society by the abuse of substances from traffic accidents, violence, and crime. Therefore, limiting a young person's substance use to alcohol as opposed to alcohol and illicit drugs would be unlikely to result in significant reductions in the consequences of substance abuse.

As long as alcohol is marketed as it is today, substance abuse prevention is like a man running a marathon with a 100 pound weight strapped to his back. There is an incredibly large and probably insurmountable burden from the beginning. When you add the pressure of the alcohol industry to minimize the focus on alcohol in our NDCS, our marathon runner has an uphill course while the course is level for the other runner, the alcohol industry. The data on use of alcohol and illicit drugs by young people shows who is winning.

Table 6.1
2004 Annual and Lifetime Use of Alcohol, Marijuana, and Illicit Drugs for 8th, 10th, and 12th Graders

	Annual	Lifetime
Any illicit drug		
8th graders	15.2	21.5
10th graders	31.1	39.8
12th graders	38.8	51.1
College	36.2	52.2
Young adults	33.7	60.5
Marijuana		
8th graders	11.8	16.3
10th graders	27.5	35.1
12th graders	34.3	45.7
College	33.3	49 1
Young adults	29.2	57.4
Alcohol		
8th graders	36.7	43.9
10th graders	58.2	64.2
12th graders	70.6	76.8
College	81.2	84.6
Young adults	84.4	89.4

Source: Johnston et al. 2005.

Experimentation

Prevention may be burdened by another weight. That is, the developmental inclination of adolescents to be sensation-seeking, rebellious, and to test the limits of authority. For example, up to now, we have only looked at the 30-day use patterns of young people to determine the extent of current use of alcohol and illicit drugs. However, annual and lifetime use of alcohol and illicit drugs provides a measure of "experimentation" by young people. Table 6.1 displays this information from the 2004 Monitoring the Future Survey.[39, 40] By 10th grade, over half of the students had used alcohol in the past year and nearly two-thirds had used alcohol sometime in their life. That increased to 7 out of 10 seniors using alcohol in the past year and over three-quarters in their life. Remember, alcohol is illegal to use for any of these young people. Close to half of 12th graders had smoked marijuana sometime in their life and over half had used an illicit drug. Clearly, experimentation with alcohol and illicit drugs is the rule rather than the exception. Therefore, prevention efforts are also meeting opposition from the desire of young people to experiment. This is not meant to condone this behavior; it is an acknowledgment of a reality.

On a positive note, as was seen in Chapter 2, illicit drug use among college students and young adults is lower than that of 12th graders. In fact, the rate of 30-day use of illicit drugs among college students and young adults is similar to the rate for 10th graders (see Tables 2.3–2.5). Therefore, it would appear that there is a "maturing" process that occurs with regard to experimentation. The same trend can be seen in annual use, although there is not as large a decrease from 12th grade to college and young adults with regard to illicit drug use. It may be that many of the 30-day users in high school reduce the frequency of their use of illicit drugs as they enter adulthood. In any case, it would appear that, in many cases, the desire of adolescents to experiment with illicit drugs begins to dissipate as they reach early adulthood.

A Pill for Every Ill

Anyone who watches television or reads magazines has noticed the tremendous number of advertisements for prescription drugs. While the use of the "purple pill" or medicine for erectile dysfunction does seem to be related to the abuse of mind-altering substances, there is an increasing attitude among Americans (assisted by heavy marketing by the pharmaceutical industry) that every problem can be solved by taking a drug. As a result, adults tend to have a variety of prescription drugs in their homes. When some of these substances are mind-altering, such as pain killers and tranquilizers, it is fairly easy for young people to gain access to these drugs through their parent's medicine cabinets. Since prescription drug use is so heavily marketed and common, young people do not tend to perceive the dangers of taking pills. Furthermore, it is difficult for parents and school personnel to detect the possession and use of these drugs by young people. There is no odor, pills are easily hidden and swallowed, and they can be mistaken for over-the-counter medications such as ibuprofen. Prescription drug use is becoming part of the social network of young people through "pharming" parties where bowls of unlabeled prescription drugs, those belonging to the participants (e.g., Ritalin) and those stolen from parents, are available for use.[41] According to national surveys, prescription drug abuse is increasing among youth and young adults. For example, there was an increase in the lifetime prevalence of nonmedical use of narcotic pain relievers from 2002 to 2004 in the 18–25 year group.[42] The Monitoring the Future survey showed increases between 2003 and 2005 in tranquilizer and OxyContin (narcotic pain reliever) use by 12th graders.[43]

Similar to the alcohol industry, the pharmaceutical industry is not motivated to take steps to limit the attractiveness or availability of its products in order to reduce the access of young people to potentially damaging medicines. For example, since 1986, the pharmaceutical industry has fought efforts to limit access to pseudoephedrine, an essential ingredient in the production of methamphetamine found in over-the-counter cold and allergy medicines.[44]

Do As I Say; Not What I Do

The "don't use drugs" message given to young people is in conflict with the behavior of many adults. When parents use alcohol excessively, take mind-altering prescription drugs for recreation, and use illegal drugs, the hypocrisy is obvious to young people and these behaviors counteract prevention efforts. Similarly, communities need to be conscious of the messages communicated to young people about alcohol use. When schools or faith-based organizations serve alcohol at social or fund-raising events, there is an implicit message regarding the need for alcohol for social interaction, recruitment of participants, and fun. There isn't anything inherently wrong about this, but communities which consistently have alcohol at events should not be surprised if their children model this behavior. If adults are not willing to inconvenience themselves a bit (i.e., have alcohol-free social events) in order to ensure that young people receive a clear message about alcohol and other drug use, all prevention efforts will have a lower probability of success.

Is There a Solution?

The many problems with substance abuse prevention that have been discussed in this chapter may lead to pessimism regarding the effort to discourage young people from using illicit drugs. However, the 30-day use data on one substance provides some guidance for the structure of an effective prevention effort. Table 2.7 shows the 30-day use of cigarettes. As was noted in Chapter 2, tobacco use (as illustrated by cigarette use) was the only substance where the target goal for 2002 was achieved and for which the 2007 goal will at least be close to being met. But, tobacco prevention has never been a focus of the NDCS. What can be learned from the effort to prevent young people from using tobacco that could be applied to substance abuse prevention in general?

First, the addiction to the drug nicotine, found in tobacco products, is clearly viewed as a public health problem in the United States. As was seen in Chapter 2, addiction to illicit drugs is perceived as a public health problem in much of the rest of the world but policies in the United States tend to treat drug use as a criminal rather than a public health problem. Second, the tremendous healthcare costs resulting from smoking motivated the states to fight the tobacco lobby. In Chapter 5, the power of the alcohol industry in blocking public policy changes was discussed. Third, the effort to prevent young people from smoking combined education about the dangers of smoking; restrictions on marketing by the tobacco industry; and policies and laws that made access to tobacco products restrictive, raised the cost of purchasing tobacco products, and limited the places where cigarette smoking was permitted. For example, when I started college in 1970, I used to buy a pack of cigarettes for 35 cents, there were cigarette vending machines, and we were allowed to smoke in class. With inflation, that pack of cigarettes would be $1.76 today.[45] In the state I attended college, a pack of cigarettes actually sells for $4.98[46] today and the campus is smoke-free. It is very difficult to even find a cigarette vending machine today.

The beginning of a concentrated, comprehensive effort to prevent young people from smoking was the passage of the Synar Amendment in 1992 (although the final implementation regulations were not disseminated until 1996). The Center for Substance Abuse Prevention oversees the implementation of the Synar Amendment which

> . . . requires states to have laws in place prohibiting the sale and distribution of tobacco products to persons under 18 and to enforce those laws effectively. States are to achieve a maximum sales-to-minors rate of not greater than 20 percent by FY 2003. CSAP has provided states with state-of-the-art materials and technical assistance to help them reach that goal. Across the Nation, States have made great strides in reducing retailer violations of the law as required by the Synar Amendment. For FY 2001, the national average retailer violation rate was 17.4 percent, down from approximately 40 percent for FY 1997. Nine States reported retailer violation rates of 10 percent or less. As a result of the successes achieved by the States in response to the Synar Amendment, the program is a true success among public health initiatives.[47]

If a state did not achieve the 20 percent sales-to-minors rate, the Block Grant funds for the state could be withheld. Remember, even though a federal agency is responsible for the oversight of the Synar Amendment, this initiative is not part of the NDCS. It was a separate law passed by Congress. Ironically, the Synar Amendment is the only demonstrably effective federal prevention effort.

Even before the Synar Amendment, states and communities were enacting laws and policies restricting smoking. However, the other major event that drove the prevention effort was the Master Tobacco Settlement Agreement of 1998.[48] This agreement, negotiated by the attorney generals of nearly every state (not the federal government), provided $260 billion in payments by tobacco companies to states over 25 years. The agreement prohibited minors from being targeted in advertisements by banning cartoon characters in ads, restricting brand-name sponsorships of events with large audiences of young people, banned outdoor advertising and youth access to free samples, and set the minimum cigarette package size at 20 (to prevent the sale of small numbers of cigarettes that would be affordable to underage smokers). A national foundation fund of $250 million over 10 years and a public education fund of $1.45 billion for 3 years were established. This money was used to start the American Legacy Foundation, which runs "truth," a youth smoking prevention campaign.[49] The Master Tobacco Settlement Agreement also required the tobacco industry to commit to reducing the access of minors to tobacco products and their consumption of cigarettes. It required the disbandment of tobacco trade associations and restricted industry lobbying.

In contrast to ONDCP's Media Campaign, research found that "truth" accounted for over one-fifth of the decline in youth smoking rates in a 3-year period.[50] The reasons why the "truth" campaign have been effective while the Media Campaign has not involves several factors. First, the tobacco industry's marketing has been restricted due to the ban on television ads and the Master Settlement Agreement.[51] The Media Campaign is, in effect, competing against alcohol because, as was discussed in Chapter 5, young people who use alcohol are much more likely to use illicit drugs than young people who do not drink. The alcohol industry, with its extensive, well-financed marketing campaign in multiple media designed to convince young people to use their product, simply overwhelms the efforts of the Media Campaign.

The "truth" campaign is also supported by a wide range of public policies that restrict access of minors to tobacco products, limit the places where people can smoke, and increase the excise taxes on tobacco products. Over the past 30 years, the American public's attitude toward smoking has definitely changed. While there have been changes in public policies with regard to alcohol (e.g., drunk driving), there is a great difference between the public's acceptance of alcohol and tobacco use.

The tobacco prevention movement has also included the mobilization of community groups in the effort. The American Legacy Web site has links to organizations in 32 states.[52] Some (but not enough) states have used tobacco settlement money to fund prevention efforts. For example, in my home state (Nevada), there is a grant competition each year for tobacco prevention and treatment proposals from community-based organizations.

The Centers for Disease Control have developed school tobacco use prevention guidelines that include the utilization of prevention curricula.[53] Although there is controversy regarding the effectiveness of school-based prevention programs in preventing any type of substance use,[54] there is some evidence that Life Skills Training, a program included on the National Registry of Evidence-based Programs and Practices, was helpful in preventing tobacco use among urban, minority students.[55]

Finally, the tobacco prevention effort included many resources to help people quit smoking. For example the American Legacy Foundation has a number of smoking cessation resources, including those targeted at pregnant women.[56] Many schools have implemented smoking cessation programs for students caught smoking on campus or for those who just want to quit.

The lessons, then, of the successful effort to reduce tobacco use by minors are that an intense public education and awareness campaign can work if, at the same time, there are limits on the "opposition's" ability to market young people to use potentially harmful, addictive substances. In addition, attitudes toward a public health problem can be changed over time with consistent messages from government agencies, combined with laws and policies that restrict access to the substance, make it expensive to purchase, and inconvenient to use.

The activities involved with the prevention of tobacco use by young people targeted universal, selective, and indicated populations and utilized nearly all of the strategies described at the beginning of this chapter. The media effort in the "truth" campaign was directed at all young people (universal). Organizations like the American Legacy Foundation targeted a specific group (e.g., pregnant women) because of a particular characteristic they share (selective). Smoking cessation programs in schools are normally targeted toward students who are caught smoking on campus (indicated). There has been information dissemination through the "truth" campaign. In addition, agencies like the American Lung Association have many informational brochures, generally distributed in medical and health clinics, hospitals, schools, and libraries. School-based programs, such as Life Skills Training, are prevention education. Community-based processes were used to mobilize groups at the local level to organize tobacco prevention efforts. Problem identification and referral strategies have been utilized when students are caught smoking on school campuses and referred to smoking cessation programs.

However, the tobacco prevention effort relied the most heavily on environmental approaches to prevention. Environmental strategies include the laws, regulations, and policies that impact the access and availability of a substance and the consequences for misusing or abusing the substance. For example, increasing the price of tobacco through excise taxes, restricting smoking in public and private locations, and enforcing laws against selling tobacco to minors have all been shown to be effective in reducing youth smoking.[57] Furthermore, environmental approaches have also proven to be effective in reducing alcohol use by young people and in decreasing alcohol-related problems. These interventions have included increasing excise taxes, raising the minimum purchase age, enforcing minimum purchase age laws through "sting" operations, zero tolerance of alcohol use by minors, lowering the blood-alcohol content for adult DUI violations, and limiting the location and density of retail alcohol outlets.[58] In fact, environmental approaches to prevention produce more rapid and significant impact on youth use of tobacco and alcohol than any other type of prevention, and these strategies enhance the other prevention efforts in place in communities.[59]

Conclusions

The title of this chapter asked the question, "Does prevention work?" Based on the results of the initiatives funded by the NDCS, the answer would be "no." However, prevention did work with regard to tobacco. We learned that a public health problem resulting from addiction could be impacted through a clear, unambiguous public policy reinforced by laws and regulations, education, and assistance for those who had trouble stopping their use.

Many people would argue that nearly the same situation exists with regard to illicit drugs. The public policy isn't quite as unambiguous since we tend to be punitive with drug abusers, but there are laws and regulations, education, and treatment for addicts. Why does one effort succeed and the other fail? The answer is alcohol.

As a society, we have to accept the fact that efforts to prevent drug use by young people can never succeed in any significant way if we won't focus our efforts on alcohol. There are data that tell us that young people who drink are much more likely to use illicit drugs than young people who do not drink. It is easy to understand that, once a young person starts to use alcohol, it is much easier for him/her to go on to try other mind-altering substances. Remember, alcohol and illicit drugs are all illegal for minors to use. Finally, based on the damage caused by alcohol, there would be minimal value in preventing young people from using illicit drugs if they used alcohol instead.

While there are efforts in the NDCS and in states to combat underage drinking, we do not have the clear, unambiguous policy that exists with regard to tobacco. We allow the alcohol industry to do a tremendous amount of marketing of their products to underage drinkers. If we won't stop this, prevention has a very low likelihood of success. If we aren't willing to enact national environmental prevention strategies (e.g., raising excise taxes and restricting retail outlets), efforts to reduce underage drinking will have limited impact. We also need a targeted, focused effort on the inappropriateness of drinking by minors to change public attitudes. The overwhelming emphasis of the NDCS on illicit drugs dilutes this focus and diverts attention from alcohol, the major substance use problem among youth.

This is not a suggestion for prohibition. People who want to smoke can still buy cigarettes and smoke them in plenty of places. It just costs more to buy the cigarettes and it is not as easy to find a place to use them. As a society, we decided that the public health hazard of cigarette smoking was so serious that it required making this legal substance expensive and more difficult to obtain and use. We simply have to decide if the public health problem of alcohol abuse, among young people and adults, is serious enough to do the same.

Some of these interventions would inconvenience and impact those who use alcohol, both moderate and heavy users. Furthermore, these changes would be strongly opposed by the alcohol industry. Therefore, our policy makers generally lack the political courage to enact these laws and regulations. If that continues to be the case, we should stop spending our money on drug prevention and just accept the reality that currently exists. The $100 plus million for the Media Campaign could be well used for addiction treatment.

The other major conclusion that can be drawn from this chapter involves the discussion about the Risk and Protective Factor theory of substance abuse prevention. It does not make much sense to categorize efforts to reduce these risk factors as "substance abuse prevention." Strategies to reduce economic deprivation, family management problems, early and persistent antisocial behavior, and so on should be much more extensive, long-lasting, and intensive than programs supported by federal substance abuse prevention dollars. Many of these "risk factors" have been present in communities and families for generations. While there certainly should be federal efforts to reduce these risk factors, they should be viewed as efforts to reduce poverty, fix urban blight, increase family stability, and improve educational and vocational competence, not as substance abuse prevention.

The activities that are currently called substance abuse prevention, such as organizing community coalitions, social skills training in schools, mentoring programs, or parenting courses, may be very beneficial. However, these activities should not be expected to prevent young people from using drugs, particularly if the risk factors are causally related to later substance abuse problems. For example, a 6-week parenting program for single mothers may help them use more effective discipline and management strategies with their children. But, if these mothers are living in poverty, in run-down neighborhoods with lots of drug use, and nothing is done about those problems, the parenting skills learned in this short time period are not going to keep these kids from using drugs. In other words, if the risk factors are also predictive of delinquency, school dropout, teen pregnancy, and violence, then substance abuse is part of a larger societal problem and substance abuse prevention should not be isolated from this reality.

Seven

Controversial Issues in Treatment

Introduction

For those who are not in the alcohol and other drugs field, their understanding of alcoholism and drug addiction and the treatment for these conditions may be based on movies, television shows, interviews with public figures who have gone through treatment, other reports in print media, or personal experiences with friends or family members. After hearing about public figures who continue to have problems with alcohol or other drugs after treatment, the public may wonder if treatment works at all. Some believe that alcoholics and drug addicts are weak individuals who deserve scorn rather than treatment. People wonder about 12-step meetings, like Alcoholics Anonymous, that seem to be like a secret club or cult.

I mentioned in Chapter 1 that I am a recovering alcoholic and drug addict. In addition, I have been a consulting psychologist for a number of treatment programs. Therefore, I have had contact, personally and professionally, with a lot of alcoholics and drug addicts. Over the years, I have been amazed at some of the recovery stories I have heard. People with criminal records, who did horrible things, turned their lives around and became productive citizens. In this field, we talk about the "miracle of recovery" to refer to the people who stop using alcohol and other drugs and lead productive lives. I can personally attest to the fact that there are many of these "miracles of recovery" in our society. I have also seen many people who have been unable to stop using alcohol and other drugs no matter how many treatment programs, religious groups, or meetings they have attended. It is important to recognize and appreciate the "miracle of recovery" and at the same time understand why many alcoholics/addicts never get there.

First, substance abuse treatment needs to be understood. Based on the popular portrayals, many people believe that the treatment process begins with a confrontation by people close to the alcoholic/addict. The alcoholic/addict then breaks down, admits his/her problem, and agrees to get help. He/she goes away to a treatment program in a quiet, rural setting, stays there for about a month, and returns "cured." Sometimes, the activities in the treatment program are depicted as a lot of group sessions that are quite confrontational and emotional. There may be some relapses along the way but, eventually, the person "gets it" and stays clean and sober.

This stereotypical illustration of substance abuse treatment is not complete fantasy. Some people are "encouraged" to seek treatment by friends and family members who are worried, scared, angry, and/or fed up. There are residential treatment programs in serene locations that last for 28 days and use a lot of group therapy. However, this is really a description of treatment for people who can afford to pay for it themselves or who have amazingly good healthcare insurance coverage. Even then, this type of residential treatment was more prevalent 5 to 10 years ago than it is today. Because of the cost, managed medical care caused a reduction in the number of residential treatment programs for those with private insurance. Furthermore, this idealized description of treatment was never the reality for the population of people who are treated in the public-sector treatment world (i.e., treatment services paid for by federal or state dollars). Since this book is about our NDCS, this discussion on treatment will be focused on the public-sector treatment arena.

Most public-sector treatment occurs in free-standing, outpatient settings (i.e., nonresidential treatment programs). In many states, treatment programs serve both public-sector clients and private pay clients (i.e., clients with medical insurance or their own financial resources).[1] Many programs may have services for special populations, such as adolescents, women with children, and clients with mental disorders in addition to a substance use disorder.[2]

Public-sector treatment also includes methadone maintenance for opiate (i.e., heroin) addicts and was described in Chapter 3. Methadone is dispensed through licensed outpatient clinics and the clients are supposed to receive counseling and support services in addition to methadone.

The services provided by treatment programs may include individual, group, and family counseling; education about addiction and related issues (e.g., HIV); social skills training (e.g., meeting nondrug using friends); and vocational, educational, financial, and self-care guidance (e.g., nutrition, hygiene). Many programs encourage or require clients to attend support group meetings, such as Alcoholics Anonymous or Narcotics Anonymous. The services provided are supposed to be designed to meet the individual needs of the clients but there is a wide variation in the quality of public-sector programs across the country. So, some programs provide the same services in the same manner to every client. There is also variation among states in the qualifications required for certification as a substance abuse counselor. While some states require at least an undergraduate degree and an extensive internship, others require only a highschool diploma or GED.

The Treatment Activities in the NDCS[3]

National Institute on Drug Abuse (NIDA)[4]

In the previous chapter, it was noted that NIDA is responsible for prevention and treatment research. In 2004 and 2005 combined, over $1 billion was spent on treatment research and over $591 million was allocated for 2006. Although NIDA has not had a PART assessment, the agency has set GPRA targets that involve the dissemination of research-based treatment approaches, materials, and strategies to community-based treatment providers and the development of medications to be used in treating addictive disorders. The dissemination targets have been met. The work on developing medications for treatment is ongoing.

Bureau of Prisons[5]

The federal prison system (part of the Department of Justice) has received slightly less than $50 million in 2004 and 2005 for treatment-related programs. A similar amount was allocated for 2006. The programs include screening and assessment of all inmates entering the federal prison system, drug abuse education, residential drug abuse treatment (treatment within specialized units), nonresiden tial drug abuse treatment (treatment integrated within the general prison system), and community transition drug abuse treatment. The latter program is a transition from residential drug abuse treatment to a community-based treatment facility following release from prison. The PART assessment rated the Bureau of Prisons programs as "moderately effective" with scores of purpose: 80, planning: 85, management: 86, and results: 75.

Office of Justice Programs[6]

This agency is part of the Department of Justice. It received over $38 million in 2004, over $64 million in 2005, and requested over $114 million in 2006 to fund two programs—Drug Courts and Residential Substance Abuse Treatment. Drug Courts, which coordinate treatment services for nonviolent offenders with drug problems as an alternative to incarceration, have been described in other chapters.

The Residential Substance Abuse Treatment program provides grants to states to operate these programs in state prison facilities. The PART assessment for Drug Courts was "results not demonstrated." It was described as, ". . . generally well-managed but faces challenges in developing outcome-oriented measures focusing on postprogram recidivism."[7] The PART scores were purpose: 100, planning: 57, management: 82, results: 53. The PART review of the Residential Substance Abuse Program also was evaluated as "results not demonstrated."[8] The scores were purpose: 60, planning, 71, management: 56, results: 20. Congress did not provide the requested funding for these programs in 2006.

Veterans Health Administration[9]

The Department of Veterans Affairs provides treatment services for veterans. The budget for this was over $402 million in 2004, $386 million in 2005, and is $401 million in 2006. No PART review has been conducted, nor has the Veterans Health Administration established outcome measures. The agency did set a target that 32 percent of the veterans served would receive appropriate care. In 2004, they determined that 28 percent had actually received appropriate care.

Substance Abuse and Mental Health Services Administration (SAMHSA)[10,11]

The Center for Substance Abuse Treatment, a part of SAMHSA, is the largest federal agency involved with treatment. The budget in 2004 and 2005 was over $1.9 billion per year with a slight decrease in 2006. The vast majority of this money is devoted to the Block Grant, over $1.4 billion each year. Most of this money is distributed to the state agency in each state responsible for the administration of substance abuse services (called the "Single State Authority"), which then distributes most of this money to community-based treatment providers to serve individuals with substance abuse problems who cannot afford treatment. The Center for Substance Abuse Treatment also has "Programs of Regional and National Significance," which generally provide competitive grants for "Best Practices" (evidenced-based practices) and "Targeted Capacity Expansion" (increasing treatment opportunities for special or underserved populations). In 2004 and 2005, the budget was about $420 million each year. In 2006, an increase of about $25 million was requested. However, this is a bit misleading. In 2004, President Bush started a program called, "Access to Recovery." Competitive grants were awarded to states to establish voucher systems in which individuals with substance abuse problems could get treatment or recovery services from providers of their choice. The idea was to allow faith-based organizations to provide these services and receive reimbursement for them. Access to Recovery was funded at about $99 million in 2004 and 2005. President Bush requested $150 million in 2006 but cut $35 million from the budget of Programs of Regional and National Significance to accommodate the increase in the Access to Recovery Program.[12] Congress did not increase the 2005 allocation for Access to Recovery in the 2006 budget but did cut the Programs of Regional and National Significance by over $23 million.

As was discussed in the previous chapter, the PART evaluation for the Block Grant was "ineffective," primarily because of the lack of uniform outcome measures. The Programs of Regional and National Significance were rated as "adequate" with scores of purpose: 80, planning: 86, management: 64, and results: 33. There was no PART assessment for any of the individual programs in this area.

From 2004 to 2006, about $9 billion will have been spent on treatment. While the PART assessments of the treatment programs are more favorable than the prevention programs discussed in Chapter 6, there is still a problem with establishing effectiveness of federally-funded treatment programs because uniform outcome measurements (i.e., establishing the effects of programs on the clients they serve) have not been implemented.

Who Is in Public-Sector Treatment? Where Does Treatment Occur?

In 2004, there were 1,870,602 admissions[13] to treatment facilities licensed or certified by the each state's Single State Authority, the agency responsible for the oversight of alcohol and other drug treatment services. Generally, those facilities that report data receive federal Block Grant dollars. Of these admissions, 69 percent were male. Sixty percent were white, over 22 percent were black, 13 percent were Hispanic, 2 percent American Indian, and 1 percent Asian/Pacific Islander. Adolescents comprised 8.5 percent of these admissions. Over three-quarters were between the ages of 20 and 49.[14]

A little over 22 percent of the admissions were for alcohol only and 18 percent were for alcohol with another drug. Heroin was the primary substance of abuse in a little more than 14 percent of the admissions, cocaine for nearly 14 percent, and methamphetamine for nearly 7 percent. Marijuana was the primary substance of abuse in nearly 16 percent of the admissions but was the primary substance of abuse in over 92 percent of the adolescent admissions. Nearly 57 percent of the clients had been admitted to treatment before; 10 percent had been admitted five or more times.[15]

The most common source of referral to treatment was the criminal justice system (36 percent). As was noted in Chapter 4, in the case of marijuana, 57 percent of the referrals were from the criminal justice system, a greater percentage than for any other substance. An individual (including self-referral) was the referral source in 34 percent of the admissions. A substance abuse provider made the referral in nearly 11 percent of the cases, another type of health care provider 7 percent, the school or an employer in 2 percent, and some other community referral source in over 10 percent of the admissions.[16]

A little more than one-fifth of the admissions were employed full-time. Over 31 percent were unemployed and nearly 40 percent were not in the workforce. Over 44 percent had at least a high school diploma or GED and a little more than one in three did not.[17] (Employment and education information is only tabulated for admissions 16 years of age and older.)

As can be seen, the admissions to public-sector treatment facilities are mostly male, nonworking, young to middle-aged adults who have been in treatment before. There are a high percentage of non-whites and relatively few are alcoholics only. The criminal justice system gets a lot of these folks into the treatment system.

Most (62.5 percent) of public-sector treatment occurs in ambulatory settings. This means that the client doesn't spend 24 hours a day in the facility. Over half of the admissions were ambulatory outpatient (1 to 2 hours, 1 to 2 days a week), nearly 11 percent were intensive outpatient (2 to 6 hours a day, 3 to 5 days a week), and almost 2 percent were detoxification (a period of abstinence from alcohol and other drugs to clear the system). Over 17 percent of admissions were in residential or rehabilitation facilities, where 24-hour care is provided. Of the admissions to residential or rehabilitation facilities, about half were short-term (less than 31 days) and about half were long-term (more than 31 days). One percent of the admissions were in a hospital. Over 20 percent of the admissions were in 24-hour service detoxification facilities.[18]

Detoxification is not really treatment. It simply is a process to get a person "cleaned up." Detoxification clients are certainly referred to treatment but many go back out on the street following detoxification. So, if you remove detoxification from the treatment data, nearly two-thirds of actual treatment occurred in an ambulatory, outpatient setting which is the least intensive treatment; nearly 13 percent in intensive outpatient, about 11 percent was short-term residential, and 11 percent was long-term residential.

Now, according to the National Institute on Drug Abuse, "Research indicates that for most patients the threshold of significant improvement is reached at about three months in treatment."[19] In other words, it takes about 90 days in treatment for meaningful progress to occur. However, when data on the discharges from treatment for 2003 is examined (see Table 7.1), only clients who completed outpatient treatment had a median length of stay that was at least 3 months (meaning 50 percent of the clients had longer stays and 50 percent had shorter stays) and less than 40 percent of outpatient clients completed treatment. None of the other types of treatment had a median length of stay that was 90 days.

Table 7.1
Discharges from Treatment and Median Length of Stay

	Completed	Transferred	Dropped Out	Terminated	Other	Median Length of Stay of Completers
Outpatient	38.3	10.1	27.9	11.4	12.4	98
Intensive outpatient	38.5	15.1	24.9	14.0	7.5	51
Short-term residential	64.1	11.4	14.6	6.5	3.4	23
Long-term residential	40.9	12.3	30.7	9.1	7.0	75
Hospital residential	68.9	15.7	10.9	3.0	1.6	15
Methadone	16.0	11.8	47.4	12.0	12.8	27

Source: Office of Applied Studies, Substance Abuse and Mental Health Services Administration. 2006. *Treatment episode data set (TEDS): 2003. Discharges from substance abuse treatment services.* DASIS Series S-30, DHHS Publication No. (SMA) 06-4139. Rockville, MD: Substance Abuse and Mental Health Services Administration.

Therefore, very few clients remained in treatment for the length of time that the National Institute on Drug Abuse recommends for "significant improvement." It can also be seen that the treatments with the longest median length of stay (outpatient, intensive outpatient, and long-term residential) all had around 40 percent of clients actually completing treatment. Nearly the same number of clients in these levels of treatment either dropped out or were terminated from treatment as completed treatment.

Effectiveness of Treatment

Based on the information in the previous section, treatment would not be expected to have much of an impact on substance use and the problems related to addiction. Surprisingly, that is not the case. The Center for Substance Abuse Treatment sponsored a congressionally mandated study of treatment outcomes for clients in public-sector treatment programs.[20] The National Treatment Improvement Evaluation Study followed 4,411 clients in 78 treatment sites across the country for 5 years. Clients were from vulnerable and underserved populations such as minorities, pregnant women, youth, public housing residents, welfare recipients, and those involved in the criminal justice system. Many of the people studied did not complete treatment, which would tend to depress any positive results. In spite of these factors, there were significant reductions in alcohol and other drug use 1 year after treatment regardless of the amount of time spent in treatment or the amount of treatment received. However, in general, stays longer than 90 days were associated with more positive treatment outcomes.[21] Positive outcomes were found in employment income, mental and physical health, criminal activity, homelessness, and high-risk behaviors for HIV infection. This study also demonstrated that the average cost savings per client in the year after treatment was $9,177, which is significantly more than the average cost of an outpatient treatment episode.[22] The savings occurred in reduced health care and crime-related costs and increased earnings by clients. Outpatient and long-term residential treatment showed the largest cost savings, but short-term residential treatment and outpatient methadone also were cost-effective.

Similar findings resulted from a study sponsored by the National Institute on Drug Abuse of 10,000 clients in nearly 100 treatment programs[23] and in a meta-analysis of 78 separate drug treatment outcome studies.[24] In addition, a summary of 51 published and 17 unpublished reports regarding the costs versus benefits of substance abuse treatment firmly validated the cost-effectiveness of treatment.[25]

The Problems

It would appear that public-sector treatment has positive effects on alcohol and other drug use and on the consequence of substance abuse and addiction. Additionally, treatment is cost-effective. These outcomes have occurred in spite of the fact that most public-sector treatment clients do not complete treatment nor do they stay in treatment long enough for the maximum benefits. Even though many federal efforts have not been able to demonstrate effectiveness for specific programs, the treatment outcome studies indicate the NDCS treatment dollars have been much better spent than the prevention dollars.

So, if clients in public-sector treatment programs are improving as a result of whatever level of services they receive, what problems exist with this situation? First, many people who need treatment do not get it. According to the results in the 2003 National Household Survey, more than 20 million people in this country needed treatment but did not get it.[26] Of course, the vast majority of those people (nearly 95 percent) did not believe they needed treatment. However, 1 million people felt they needed treatment but did not get it.[27] The reasons given by these people were—not ready to stop using (41 percent), cost/insurance barriers (33 percent), the stigma of alcohol and drug problems (nearly 20 percent), able to handle the problem without treatment (17 percent), access barriers other than cost, such as lack of child care (12 percent), did not know where to go (nearly 9 percent).[28] (The percentages add up to more than 100 percent because more than one reason could be given). Certainly, if a person isn't ready to stop using alcohol or other drugs or thinks he or she can handle the problem on his or her own, that's not a problem the government can solve. However, cost/insurance and access barriers are clearly related to money/resources. For example, a single parent cannot leave children alone while he or she goes to treatment. Stigma may not seem to be related to government policies, but, as was discussed in Chapter 3, the United States treats the possession and use of illicit drugs as a criminal rather than a public health problem. That type of attitude would not tend to encourage those people with illicit drug problems to seek treatment. Finally, people who need and want treatment are generally quite vulnerable and fragile at the time they are trying to find a treatment program. If it is not easy to locate treatment resources, their motivation to get in a treatment program may be easily discouraged. Therefore, state agencies must make it as simple as possible to locate public-sector treatment.

Other problems relate to the retention of clients in treatment and the length of treatment. In any earlier section, it was noted that only about 40 percent of outpatient clients complete treatment. Furthermore, most clients are not in programs that last the 90 days recommended by the National Institute on Drug Abuse. The latter problem is related to resources. Many states do not have enough money to fund public-sector programs so that the programs can last 90 days or more. The Block Grant and state funds simply do not go far enough. The retention of clients in programs is much more complex. Clients may believe they are "cured" and leave. They can become uncomfortable with a sober lifestyle and leave. The client may have other problems in addition to alcohol and other drug use that cannot be addressed in the treatment program. The client's treatment program may be managed inappropriately because of poor staff training or lack of knowledge and, therefore, the client becomes dissatisfied and leaves. The Center for Substance Abuse Treatment has implemented some initiatives to improve the retention of clients in treatment but this problem is difficult to overcome.

Finally, most clients who are in treatment do not remain abstinent from alcohol and other drugs. Earlier in the chapter, it was noted that nearly 57 percent of public-sector clients had more than one treatment admission. A literature review revealed that 40 percent to 60 percent of clients who were treated for dependence on alcohol, cocaine, or heroin were continually abstinent for 1 year following treatment. [29] An additional 15 percent to 30 percent used alcohol or other drugs in a nondependent manner (this finding will be discussed in more detail later in the chapter). The best predictors of relapse were low socioeconomic status, the presence of a co-occurring mental disorder, and lack of family and social support systems.

There are simple solutions to some of the problems mentioned in this section. Clearly, additional resources would allow treatment programs to increase the length of time clients are engaged in treatment and would help remove some of the barriers that exist for people who want to enter treatment. A greater effort on public awareness would help people who want treatment locate available treatment resources.

The problem of stigma is more complex. As has been said, stigma is partially related to government policies that treat drug addiction as a criminal rather than a public health problem. However, stigma is also a result of public stereotypes of alcoholics and drug addicts. Fortunately, there is a growing movement to combat the stigma of addiction organized by groups of recovering alcoholics and drug addicts, their family members, and public allies.[30]

The other problems mentioned in this section (the fact that so many people with alcohol and other drug problems do not acknowledge the need for help, the problem of retaining clients in treatment, and the frequency of relapse among clients following treatment) are related to each other. In order to understand this relationship, it is necessary to examine some controversial issues in treatment.

Is Alcoholism/Addiction a Disease?

Many people view alcoholism/addiction as a result of voluntary behavior that is seen as sinful from a moral/religious perspective or irresponsible from a secular point of view.

However, in 1960, E. M. Jellinek presented an argument that alcoholism was a medical disease.[31] Following Jellinek's work, the American Psychiatric Association began to use the term "disease" to describe alcoholism and the American Medical Association followed in 1966.[32] As with many concepts and theoretical models in this field, the disease concept was originally applied to alcoholism and has been generalized to addiction to other drugs.

In the disease concept of alcoholism/addiction, the condition is viewed as a primary disease. That is, it is not caused by another condition (e.g., depression or family problems). The disease is progressive, with predictable stages including a loss of control over drinking and/or drug use. In addition, the disease of alcoholism/addiction is chronic (continues for life), and it is incurable. In this conceptualization of the disease concept, the only justifiable goal is abstinence from alcohol and illicit drugs.

The disease concept is associated with Alcoholics Anonymous and Narcotics Anonymous.[33] Furthermore, the most widely emulated approach to treatment, the Minnesota Model developed by the Hazeldon Foundation, incorporates the disease concept of alcoholism/addiction in its treatment program.[34]

In the late 1980s, books were published that criticized the disease concept of alcoholism, primarily due to the lack of evidence that all alcoholics/addicts lost control of their use of alcohol and other drugs in all instances, some people classified as alcoholics/addicts returned to moderate levels of use, and the stages of the disease did not seem to follow a predictable sequence with many people.[35]

Is Alcoholism/Addiction a Chronic Medical Condition?

While the traditional view of the disease concept is still prevalent in many treatment programs, recent work has conceptualized alcoholism/addiction as a chronic medical condition rather than as a disease.[36] The difference is more than semantic. While disease concept proponents attempt to describe a unique set of progressive stages of the disease of addiction, those who prefer a conceptualization of addiction as a chronic medical condition establish their argument on the basis of the similarity of alcohol and other drug dependence to other chronic medical conditions, such as diabetes, hypertension, and asthma. For example, medical scholars in the field have shown that the genetic heritability and the relapse rate for alcoholism/addiction are similar to these other chronic medical conditions. The major implication in conceptualizing alcoholism/addiction as a chronic medical condition is that treatment requires continuing care. An article on this topic uses an analogy with regard to hypertension to illustrate the lack of logic with regard to the current way substance abuse treatment is provided:

> Hypertensive patients would be admitted to a 28-day hypertension rehabilitation program, where they would receive group and individual counseling regarding behavioral control of diet, exercise, and lifestyle. Very few would be prescribed medications, since the prevailing insurance restrictions would discourage maintenance medications. Patients completing the program would be discharged to community resources, typically without continued medical monitoring. An evaluation of these patients 6 to 12 months following discharge would count as successes only those who had remained continuously normotensive for the entire postdischarge period.[37]

In other words, if addiction is a chronic medical condition, noncompliance with prescribed treatment and relapse is expected in a large number of patients. Treatment progress should be measured on the extent of compliance with the treatment plan rather than as a success/failure dichotomy. Furthermore, for an extended period of time, there should be periodic monitoring of treatment compliance, and the treatment plan should be modified as needed.

For many people, the difficulty with viewing alcohol or other drug dependence as a chronic medical condition is the voluntary action involved in taking alcohol or other drugs. However, voluntary action is a factor in the development of many chronic medical conditions. You may have a genetic predisposition for hypertension but becoming obese and smoking are causal factors in the development of the condition, both of which are voluntary behaviors. There are also individual differences in the pleasurable response that people have to alcohol and other drugs. Those that experience more pleasure are more likely to repeat the behaviors. There is evidence that these differences in pleasurable responses are genetic.[38] Therefore, those individuals whose genetic predisposition allows them to experience maximum pleasure from alcohol and other drugs are the most likely to use substances the most frequently and to subsequently develop substance abuse problems. While it is still a voluntary action to use alcohol and other drugs, it is far easier for someone who does not experience a great deal of pleasure from alcohol and other drugs to limit their use.

Treatment for Individuals with Co-occurring Mental Disorders

According to the Center for Substance Abuse Treatment, more than 1 in 5 adults (8 million Americans) with a substance abuse or dependence disorder also were diagnosed with a serious mental illness in the past year. Over half of those with a lifetime alcohol abuse or dependence disorder also had a serious mental illness in their lifetime. This figure rose to nearly 60 percent for those with an illicit drug abuse or dependence disorder and was over 70 percent for people with alcohol and illicit drug disorders.[39] This is important because over two-thirds of clients in treatment for a substance use disorder were treated in facilities whose primary focus was substance abuse services[40] and public-sector treatment programs have normally not been equipped to provide appropriate services for clients with co-occurring mental disorders. The clinical staff in public-sector treatment programs consist of mostly drug and alcohol counselors who are not qualified or licensed to provide other mental health services. While programs might have consultants who are psychiatrists, psychologists, clinical social workers, or other licensed mental health professionals, most programs cannot afford to have these clinicians on staff full time. Therefore, clients receive substance abuse treatment but, if their other mental disorder is diagnosed, the client has to be referred elsewhere for treatment of the co-occurring mental disorder.

A common example might illustrate how this could cause problems in the treatment of clients. A woman in a treatment program suffers from posttraumatic stress disorder due to repeated instances of childhood sexual abuse (researchers have found that nearly three-quarters of women in treatment have a history of sexual abuse).[41] As she progresses in treatment, the woman begins to experience the negative emotional states associated with posttraumatic stress disorder (e.g., anxiety, panic, agitation). In the past, she has used alcohol and other drugs to manage these negative emotions. If the treatment staff are not trained and qualified to treat her posttraumatic stress disorder, the client will have no other resources to manage her negative emotions. The probability of this client remaining abstinent from alcohol and other drugs is low.

According to the Center for Substance Abuse Treatment, nearly 12 percent of substance abuse treatment clients had a lifetime diagnosis of major depressive disorder, almost 4 percent had a generalized anxiety disorder, and over 39 percent had a diagnosis of antisocial personality disorder. Amazingly, nearly 60 percent of individuals who used a combination of cocaine, heroin, and alcohol were diagnosed with antisocial personality disorder.[42] Since antisocial personality disorder is so pervasive among clients in treatment for a substance use disorder, this condition will be discussed in detail.

The *Diagnostic and Statistical Manual of Mental Disorders*, the reference book used by mental health professionals for diagnosis, reports that the prevalence of antisocial personality disorder in the general population is about 3 percent for men and 1 percent for women,[43] so the percentages with this condition among the substance abuse treatment population are astounding. According to the American Psychiatric Association, antisocial personality disorder is defined as

... a pervasive pattern of disregard for and violation of the rights of others occurring since age 15 years, as indicated by three (or more) of the following:

1. failure to conform to social norms with respect to lawful behaviors as indicated by repeatedly performing acts that are grounds for arrest

2. deceitfulness, as indicated by repeated lying, use of aliases, or conning others for personal profit or pleasure

3. impulsivity or failure to plan ahead

4. irritability and aggressiveness, as indicated by repeated physical fights or assaults

5. reckless disregard for safety of self or others

6. consistent irresponsibility, as indicated by repeated failure to sustain consistent work behavior or honor financial obligations

7. lack of remorse, as indicated by being indifferent to or rationalizing having hurt, mistreated, or stolen from another[44]

Based on these criteria, it is clear that people with antisocial personality disorder would be unpleasant to deal with and might be frightening. It should also be pointed out that mental disorders such as depression and anxiety can often be of relatively short duration (6 months to several years). In contrast, a personality disorder is, by definition, an enduring pattern of behavior that has been present since adolescence or early adulthood and rarely, if ever, changes.

A study by NIDA researchers confirmed the high rate of antisocial personality disorder among clients with substance use disorders and hypothesized that substance use disorders and antisocial personality disorders both are associated with impaired development of certain brain structures that guide high-level decision making.[45]

The importance of this information on antisocial personality disorder involves the treatment and prognosis for the most commonly diagnosed co-occurring mental disorders. Depressive disorders and anxiety disorders can be well-managed with therapy and medications. Here is what experts say about antisocial personality disorder: "... unresponsive to most therapeutic interventions ... self-help groups, such as AA; and even marriage to a person as needy as the patient—all seem to be more useful to the antisocial personality than one-to-one therapy."[46] "No medications are routinely used or specifically approved for ASP (antisocial personality disorder) treatment. Several drugs, however, have been shown to reduce aggression—a common problem for many antisocials ... Incarceration may be the best way to control the most severe and persistent cases of antisocial personality disorder."[47] "Antisocial personality disorder is considered one of the most difficult of all personality disorders to treat. Individuals rarely seek treatment on their own and may only initiate therapy when mandated by a court. The efficacy of treatment for antisocial personality disorder is largely unknown."[48]

The problem is obvious. The most frequent co-occurring mental disorder among substance abuse clients is antisocial personality disorder, a condition that is basically untreatable by the methods available to most mental health professionals. If nearly 4 in 10 clients have this condition, alcohol and drug abuse counselors in public-sector treatment programs are going to have limited success simply because a large portion of their treatment population has antisocial personality disorder.

Abstinence

Earlier in the chapter, a result from a literature review was cited that found that 15–30 percent of clients who had been in treatment were using alcohol and/or other drugs in a "nondependent" manner.[49] This means that those clients are using mind-altering substances moderately, just like people who do not need treatment. This finding is contradictory to the precepts of the disease concept and is in opposition to any treatment philosophy I have ever heard in a public-sector treatment program. Clients are told that they can never drink or use drugs again and, if they do, they will end up in the same place (or worse) than before they entered treatment.

So, how can it be that a sizeable number of former clients are using alcohol and other drugs moderately? Perhaps they were not diagnosed correctly when they entered treatment. That is certainly possible, particularly in referrals from the criminal justice system, schools, or from employers. Individuals may be coerced to enter treatment by these entities based on evidence of an alcohol or other drug problem. The individual may want to reduce pressure from the court, school, or employer by agreeing to enter treatment and the treatment program may not do a thorough assessment and diagnosis. Furthermore, there is evidence that some individuals with mild to moderate problems with alcohol are able to develop nonproblematic drinking patterns.[50] Perhaps the 15–30 percent that are drinking or using drugs in a nondependent manner should have been diagnosed differently. Of course, the possibility cannot be dismissed that some proportion of clients properly diagnosed with a substance dependent disorder use alcohol or other drugs nonproblematically later in life.

Chronic Addiction

Earlier in the chapter, it was noted that nearly 57 percent of clients in public-sector treatment had been in treatment previously and 10 percent had been admitted to treatment five or more times.[51] Certainly, if addiction is a chronic medical condition, it would not be surprising to find that alcoholics/addicts had multiple treatment episodes. However, five or more times implies a chronic addiction problem that simply is not responding to treatment. Also, everyone has seen chronic alcoholics/addicts on the street in urban areas and many of these individuals die (from a variety of causes) without ever becoming clean and sober. In fact, a government study found that 38 percent of the homeless had an alcohol problem and another 26 percent had a drug problem.[52]

In the late 1990s the NDCSs in the Clinton administration did emphasize the treatment of chronic addicts, recognizing that this population was responsible for a large proportion of illegal drug consumption, crime-related drug use, and other health problems (e.g., HIV). However, the treatment of chronic addicts has not been a focus in the NDCSs of the Bush administration. Needless to say, those individuals who have been in treatment numerous times and/or are homeless and/or have multiple contacts with the criminal justice system are very difficult to treat. The question is, "Can they be helped?"

12-Step Programs and Spirituality

The final controversial issue in treatment to be discussed involves programs such as Alcoholics Anonymous and Narcotics Anonymous that utilize the 12-steps to recovery as their core element. These programs are spiritual in nature, with references to a Higher Power that can be God or any other conceptualization that fits for the individual. The emphasis on spirituality for recovery is quite unique in a health-related field. As can be imagined, this inspires controversy and misunderstanding, with some people believing that 12-step programs are secret cults that brainwash participants into believing that they are not responsible for their behavior.

Alcoholics Anonymous (AA) began 70 years ago and now has over 15 million people participating in over 500,000 groups worldwide.[53] Other groups, such as Narcotics Anonymous, Gamblers Anonymous, and Al-Anon (for family members of alcoholics/addicts) developed later and were modeled on the principles of AA. Many treatment programs utilize the 12-steps of recovery, particularly the first three steps, in treatment and may strongly encourage or require attendance at 12-step meetings. Meetings are free and run by members. Donations from members maintain meeting rooms and an organizational structure. AA does not allow donations from any outside entities or organizations. You become a member of AA simply by showing up at a meeting and by having a desire to stop drinking or using drugs (AA is not limited to alcoholics). If a person relapses, he or she is welcomed back the next time.

The 12-steps of recovery will not be restated here. They are available from the AA Web site (www.alcoholics-anonymous.org). However, it should be noted that only the first and last steps mention "alcohol." The steps are actually a suggestion for thinking and living that involve acceptance, forgiveness, humility, and service to others. In that sense, the 12-steps of recovery can be helpful for addicts and nonaddicts alike.

A professional work group was formed by the Substance Abuse and Mental Health Services Administration to investigate the effectiveness of self-help groups. Based on a review of the literature, the group concluded that

- Longitudinal studies associate Alcoholics Anonymous and Narcotics Anonymous participation with greater likelihood of abstinence, improved social functioning, and greater self-efficacy. Participation seems more helpful when members engage in other group activities in addition to attending meetings.

- Twelve-step self-help groups significantly reduce health care utilization and costs, removing a significant burden from the health care system.

- Self-help groups are best viewed as a form of continuing care rather than as a substitute for acute treatment services (e.g., detoxification, hospital-based treatment, etc.).

- Randomized trials with coerced populations suggest that AA combined with professional treatment is superior to AA alone.[54]

The controversy about 12-step groups generally involves the issue of spirituality, especially when 12-step meetings are mandated by a treatment program or the court. This can be perceived as forcing an individual to accept a religious orientation in spite of the individual's personal beliefs. While 12-step meetings have no particular religious affiliation or philosophy, God is regularly mentioned and the Lord's Prayer is recited at AA meetings. Therefore, it is certainly understandable how atheists or those with a religious philosophy different than Christianity might feel uncomfortable. While there are support groups that do not have a spiritual orientation, these groups are far less numerous than AA. Therefore, people mandated to attend a support group for alcoholics or addicts may have very little choice except AA or NA.

Some people have also perceived that the 12-step movement encourages people to shift responsibility for their problems to external forces. The first of the 12 steps of AA is "We admitted we were powerless over alcohol—that our lives had become unmanageable." The AA philosophy does encourage a belief that alcoholics/addicts are powerless over alcohol and illicit drugs, once they ingest these substances. However, the AA program is about personal responsibility. The decision to drink or use drugs is completely within a member's control. Furthermore, AA philosophy does teach that alcoholics/addicts are responsible for their actions while they were drinking and drugging. In fact, the 12 steps include making amends to all people harmed by the member's drinking and drug use. Twelve-step and other spiritual support programs clearly can assist in the recovery process for many alcoholics and addicts. If addiction is seen as a chronic medical condition that requires ongoing support to maintain lifestyle changes, groups such as AA are very important since most people do not have the resources for long-term professional services. However, since 12-step groups have a spiritual orientation, this type of support may not be appropriate for every alcoholic/addict.

Relationship of the Problems to the Controversial Issues

To understand how the problems of so many people not acknowledging a substance abuse problem, the failure to retain people in treatment, and the frequency of relapse relate to the controversial issues that have been discussed, examples of real people will be used. I have known each of these people either by family relationship, professional relationship, or my own recovery experience. All the names are fabricated.

Herbert: This white, Jewish man was a maintenance drinker. That is, he drank alcoholically for many years but was rarely drunk. He kept a certain amount of alcohol in his body most of the time. Herbert was married for over 50 years and self-employed successfully for that time. When he was 60, he had to start taking a medicine that affected his liver. The doctor told him he could not drink. He stopped drinking immediately, without treatment and with no withdrawal symptoms, and never drank again for the next 19 years that he lived. He died of unrelated causes. (maintenance drinker)[55]

Lonnie: A Hispanic/American Indian, Lonnie was a heroin addict at age 25. After time in a federal prison for drug trafficking, he entered a residential, faith-based treatment program that lasted 1 year. Lonnie became a born-again Christian, worked for the treatment program, and eventually became a treatment director. Today, Lonnie is an upstanding citizen and politically well connected. He drinks alcohol moderately. (faith-based heroin addict)

Rachel: This white woman with two DUIs and a possession of cocaine charge was court-ordered to go to AA or NA and counseling. Rachel was very intelligent but diagnosed with antisocial personality disorder. She hated AA, claiming that she was an atheist. While she was in counseling, Rachel was arrested for her third DUI and sent to prison. (antisocial cocaine abuser)

Raymond: Raymond was a classic alcoholic. A white male, he was hiding bottles everywhere and drinking constantly by the age of 55. His liver was nearly destroyed when his family forced him to get help. He went to a treatment program that used aversive conditioning. That is, the treatment program provided him with alcohol but also gave him a substance that made him extremely nauseous when he drank. The treatment lasted about 3 weeks. Raymond never drank again and never attended any type of self-help group. He died at age 67 of lung cancer. (nausea-treatment alcoholic)

Cheryl: This white woman has been a heroin addict for many years. She comes from an intact, supportive family. Cheryl has been in methadone programs, faith-based programs, and traditional treatment programs. However, she continues to use heroin. (relapsing heroin user)

Fred: An African-American man, Fred was briefly jailed following a DUI when he was 45. Fred used alcohol and marijuana. He was ordered to attend DUI school and a few AA meetings. After going to AA, Fred realized he was alcoholic.

He voluntarily entered a traditional 28-day treatment program. Twenty-five years later, he attends AA meetings regularly and has never had a drink or used marijuana in all these years. (DUI/AA)

As these few examples illustrate, there is tremendous variability in every aspect of alcoholism/addiction and substance abuse treatment, including gender, religion, and race. At various times, any of these people might have said that they had an alcohol or other drug problem but did not think they needed help. That is not unusual or surprising. The lifestyle changes required when a person has a substance abuse problem are difficult. Most of us know how hard it is to change our diet and exercise patterns. Many people would say "yes" if asked whether they were overweight but "no" if asked whether they wanted to go on a diet and exercise more to lose weight. Imagine the magnitude of this difficulty when a person has a physical and/or psychological dependence on alcohol or other drugs. So, it is no shock that 19 million Americans say they have a substance abuse problem but that they do not need help. Raymond (nausea-treatment alcoholic), Fred (DUI/AA), and Cheryl (relapsing heroin user) perfectly fit the disease concept of addiction. However, Fred is the only one who entered recovery in the traditional manner, through a disease concept treatment program and AA. Raymond stayed sober after a stay in a nontraditional treatment program and without ever attending AA. Cheryl has been in numerous treatment programs, faith-based, methadone, and traditional, and continues to relapse in spite of having a great family support system.

Does the chronic medical condition concept make sense? Again, it does for some of the people in our example. Certainly, the disease model examples (Raymond, Fred, Cheryl) appear to have chronic medical conditions. However, Raymond (nausea-treatment alcoholic) did not have any continuing care after treatment, yet he remained sober. Herbert (maintenance drinker) certainly had a chronic problem with alcohol. But, he never had any formal treatment intervention for his drinking and was able to stop drinking and never start again without any assistance.

Rachel (antisocial cocaine abuser) had the most common co-occurring mental disorder, antisocial personality disorder, and, predictably, she failed to adhere to a treatment program and ended up in prison. When you read the criteria for antisocial personality disorder, it is no surprise that individuals with this condition gravitate toward the heavy use of alcohol and other drugs. The nature of the disorder combined with the heavy use of alcohol and other drugs is certainly going to lead to problems. No doubt, addiction to alcohol and other drugs may result. However, it may not make sense to conceptualize clients with antisocial personality disorder as having either a "disease" or a "chronic medical condition." While the NIDA researchers may be correct that there are similarities in brain development between addicts and antisocial personality disorder, this has little practical utility in the treatment of this population. If the client with antisocial personality disorder does quit using alcohol and other drugs, what do you have? You have a sober individual with antisocial personality disorder. I still would not want this person as a neighbor. However, the likelihood is that clients with antisocial personality disorder drop out of treatment or, if forced to remain in treatment by an authority like the court, relapse soon after completing treatment. This would help partially explain the high percentage of clients who terminate treatment and who relapse.

The issue of abstinence (or lack of) is quite complex. Raymond (nausea-treatment alcoholic), Fred (DUI/AA), and Herbert (maintenance drinker) all stayed abstinent from alcohol but through very different processes. Cheryl (relapsing heroin user) and Rachel (antisocial cocaine abuser) returned to problematic use of alcohol and other drugs and would be called "treatment failures." What about Lonnie (faith-based heroin addict)? His treatment program was faith-based. It did not utilize 12-steps or AA but it did require abstinence. Most people in this field would predict that Lonnie's alcohol use would lead to a return to heroin or result in the development of an alcohol problem. However, this has not happened. He seems to be one of the 15–30 percent of clients who uses alcohol or other drugs moderately following treatment. Again, this suggests that it is not possible to categorize all clients with diagnosed substance use disorders in the same manner.

Cheryl (relapsing heroin user) and Rachel (antisocial cocaine abuser) can be called "chronic addicts" but for very different reasons. Rachel has antisocial personality disorder. Why can't Cheryl recover? I don't know. Maybe she will someday or maybe she will die from this addiction.

Finally, if you asked Fred (DUI/AA) what saved his life, he will tell you AA. Personally, I know many people who would say the same thing. But, Raymond (nausea-treatment alcoholic), Herbert (maintenance drinker), and Lonnie (faith-based heroin addict) got better without AA. So, AA is not the only way.

Conclusions

Even though federal treatment initiatives cannot demonstrate effectiveness, there is evidence that public-sector treatment has benefits and is cost-effective. There is a need for additional resources so that those who need and want treatment can get it and treatment will be of sufficient length for maximum effectiveness. In addition, the fact that so many clients leave treatment early and so many relapse raises questions about how treatment can be improved. Additionally, there are controversial issues in the field that have an impact on treatment.

From the evidence that has been discussed, alcoholism/addiction is clearly a heterogeneous condition. It probably has many causes, can be treated in many ways, and has a variety of different outcomes. It is no surprise that many people don't want to change their alcohol and other drug use because the lifestyle changes required are difficult. In order to find an explanation as to why so many people leave treatment early and so many people relapse, the percentage of clients with antisocial personality disorder would be a good place to start. For the remainder of clients in treatment, the notion of a chronic medical condition would suggest that treatment needs to be longer and some type of continuing care or contact is required. That could be AA, the advantages being it is free, readily available, provides a support group, and encourages a positive approach to thinking and living. However, there are other alternatives. As the examples illustrated, there are many different paths to recovery from alcoholism and addiction. Some people get sober on their own. Some have a religious experience through a faith-based organization or institution. Clients with heroin addiction may free themselves from this drug through the use of methadone. Other people with substance abuse problems may find a solution through support groups that have a very different philosophy than AA. With all of the possible roads to recovery, the current Administration's Access to Recovery initiative, mentioned earlier in this chapter, makes sense. This program would allow people with substance abuse problems to access treatment and recovery programs that meet their needs and philosophy. Certainly, everyone with a substance use disorder should be given chances to recover from addiction. The question is, how many chances?

Just like any other condition, there will be those who do not succeed in treatment, in spite of satisfactory care, good support systems, and adequate resources. The question must be raised as to whether it makes sense to continually provide resources for those who repeatedly cannot or will not maintain compliance with treatment recommendations.

Eight

Can the Supply Ever Be Stopped?

Introduction

The cover of *Newsweek* magazine on August 8, 2005, was "The Meth Epidemic: Inside America's New Drug Crisis." The Bush administration seemed to agree as Drug Czar John Walters, Attorney General Alberto Gonzales, and Health and Human Services Secretary Mike Leavitt toured facilities and programs in Tennessee on August 18, 2005, to highlight the government's efforts to combat methamphetamine.[1] Many of the initiatives involve laws to restrict the acquisition of psuedoephedrine, a precursor ingredient in the manufacture of methamphetamine found in over-the-counter cold medications. However, Congressional members have criticized the initiatives as inadequate, as there are loopholes that will still allow people to acquire large amounts of psuedoephedrine.[2] In addition, restrictions on purchasing quantities of psuedoephedrine do not exist in Mexico. So it is relatively easy to bring this substance into the United States.

Since the beginning of the War on Drugs, the United States has focused, at various times, on powder cocaine, crack (smokeable cocaine), heroin, marijuana, LSD, ecstasy, OxyContin (a prescription pain medication), and now methamphetamine. In each case, significant resources have been allocated to reducing the supply of the targeted drug in this country by destroying the source of the drugs here and abroad (eradication), disrupting efforts to bring the drugs to market in the United States (interdiction), and arresting those who distribute the drugs (domestic law enforcement). As was seen in Chapter 2, these efforts have not had any impact on the price, purity, or availability of illegal drugs in this country. This is certainly not the result of a lack of resources devoted to this cause. More than $7.7 billion was provided for supply reduction in fiscal year 2006, 62 percent of the total NDCS budget.[3] With all of this money for supply reduction and the lack of results, some explanation is required. Perhaps the types of activities to disrupt the supply of illegal drugs are inappropriate. Or, perhaps the goal is impossible. Both of these possibilities will be discussed in this chapter. First, there will be a discussion of what the federal government is currently doing to reduce the supply of illegal drugs.

The Major Supply Reduction Activities in the NDCS[4]

Bureau of International Narcotics and Law Enforcement Affairs[5]

This State Department agency has a budget of between $900 million and $1.0 billion a year from 2004 to 2006 for two programs: International Narcotics Control & Law Enforcement (INCLE) and Andean Counterdrug Initiative (ACI). INCLE programs

> . . . focus on reducing the amount of illegal drugs entering the United States by targeting drugs both at the source and in-transit. Programs are designed to reduce drug cultivation through enforcement, eradication, and alternative development; strengthen the capacity of law enforcement institutions to investigate and prosecute major drug trafficking organizations; improve the capacity of host national police and military forces to attack narcotics production and trafficking centers; and foster regional and global cooperation against drug trafficking.[6]

In the 2006 budget request, over half of the INCLE funds were devoted to Afghanistan, mainly for eradication of poppy fields.

The goals of the ACI are

> . . . to reduce and disrupt the flow of drugs to the United States, assist host country efforts to eradicate drug crops, stop the transportation of drugs and illicit proceeds within and outside of these countries, and in the case of Colombia support a Colombian campaign to battle narco-terrorism in its national territory.[7]

Nearly two-thirds of the 2006 budget request for ACI was devoted to Colombia for coca and poppy eradication and disruption of drug trafficking.

The PART assessment rated both programs as "adequate." Both programs received perfect scores of 100 for purpose. However, the scores for the results of these programs were 34 for ACI and 33 for INCLE. In other words, the programs have clearly defined goals but there is not much evidence that the goals are being achieved. That is an interesting definition of "adequate."

Department of Defense[8]

The Department of Defense received $803 million in FY 2006, compared to $1 billion in 2005 and $836 million in 2004. Most of this money was for international support to ". . . detect, interdict, disrupt or curtail activities related to substances, material, weapons or resources used to finance, support, secure, cultivate, process or transport illegal drugs."[9] There is no PART assessment for the Department of Defense supply reduction activities.

Homeland Security[10]

There are three agencies in the Department of Homeland Security involved with supply reduction. The United States Coast Guard, with a 2006 budget of over $1 billion ($200 million more than in 2004 and $130 million more than in 2005) for interdiction ". . . to reduce the flow of illegal drugs entering the United States by denying smugglers their maritime routes."[11] The PART assessment was "results not demonstrated," with a results score of 25. However, the Coast Guard did get a perfect 100 for purpose. The budget for the Immigration and Customs Enforcement (ICE) has gone from nearly $575 million in 2004 to $362 million in 2005 and $437 million in 2006. The decrease from 2004 to 2005 was the transfer of interdiction activities to Customs and Border Protection. Nearly all of the ICE funding is devoted to investigations ". . . to enforce the regulations concerning the movement of carriers, persons, and commodities between the United States and other nations, which enables ICE to play a key role in the overall antidrug effort with a nexus to the border."[12] The investigations involve money laundering and the interdiction of large amounts of currency. There has not been a PART assessment of the drug component for ICE. Customs and Border Protection's drug-related budget has increased from a little over $1 billion in 2004 to nearly $1.6 billion in 2006, mainly because of enhanced interdiction activities. The Customs and Border Protection agency ". . . has implemented aggressive border enforcement strategies that are designed to interdict and disrupt the flow of narcotics and ill-gotten gains across the nation's borders and dismantle the related smuggling organizations."[13] There has not been a PART assessment of the drug component of Customs and Border Protection.

Department of Justice[14]

There are three agencies in the Department of Justice with activities in the supply reduction area. The Office of Justice Programs has some responsibilities in this area, including a regional information system to assist state and local law enforcement, funding for local prosecutor offices in the four states along the U.S./Mexican border, methamphetamine enforcement and cleanup, and domestic marijuana eradication. There has not been a PART assessment for any of these programs. The total supply reduction funding in the Office of Justice Programs was nearly $172 million in 2004, nearly $186 million in 2005, and $188 million in 2006.

The second Department of Justice entity, the Organized Crime Drug Enforcement Task Force (OCDETF)

> ... was established in 1982 as a multi-agency partnership among federal, state and local law enforcement officers and prosecutors, working side by side, to identify, dismantle and disrupt sophisticated national and international drug trafficking and money laundering organizations ... The OCDETF program identifies, disrupts and dismantles major drug supply and money laundering organizations through coordinated, nationwide investigations targeting the entire infrastructure of these enterprises—from the foreign-based suppliers, to the domestic transportation and smuggling systems, to the regional and local distribution networks and the financial operations.[15]

The OCDETF supply reduction budget was nearly $550 million in 2004 and $554 million in 2005. The 2006 budget was reduced to $483 million because certain functions were transferred to other departments. There has been no PART assessment. Finally, the Department of Justice includes the Drug Enforcement Administration (DEA) whose budget was $1.7 billion in 2004, nearly $1.8 billion in 2005, and almost $1.9 billion in 2006. DEA's mission is to

> ... enforce the controlled substances laws and regulations of the United States and bring to the criminal and civil justice system of the United States, or any other competent jurisdiction, those organizations and principal members of organizations involved in the growing, manufacturing, or distribution of controlled substances appearing in or destined for illicit traffic in the United States; and to support non-enforcement programs aimed at reducing the availability of illicit controlled substances on the domestic and international markets.[16]

The DEA's PART assessment was "adequate" with a perfect score of 100 for purpose, very high scores in planning and management, and a 25 in results. The DEA appears to be a well run organization with a clear direction that cannot demonstrate its effectiveness.

In summary, the federal agencies involved with supply reduction are engaged in many activities in the areas of intelligence gathering, interdiction, investigations, and prosecution here and abroad. The operations often require military equipment and high technology. The agencies involved have well-defined goals and are managed efficiently. However, in no instance in which an independent evaluation was conducted, could any of these agencies show that their activities produced results. The PART assessments are not surprising since, as was discussed in Chapter 2, no NDCS targets have been achieved in the supply reduction area.

Are the Supply Reduction Activities in the NDCS Inappropriate?

In the 2005 NDCS, the rationale for the type of activities the United States employs to reduce the supply of illegal drugs is explained:

> The strategy of the U.S. Government is to disrupt the market for illegal drugs—and to do so in a way that both reduces the profitability of the drug trade and increases the costs of drugs to consumers. In other words, we seek to inflict on this business what every legal business fears—escalating costs, diminishing profits, and unreliable suppliers. But how do we disrupt a market whose profits seem limitless? First, it is important to understand that the drug trade is not in fact limitlessly profitable. Like every other business, the supply of and demand for illegal drugs exist in equilibrium; there is a price beyond which customers, particularly young people, will not pay for drugs. It follows that, when supplies are disrupted, prices go up, or drug supplies become erratic. Prices rising too much can precipitate a crisis for the individual user, encouraging an attempt at drug treatment. Use, in turn, goes down. Many drug trafficking organizations are complex, far-flung international businesses, often compared to multinational corporations. Yet others have more in common with the vast numbers of small networked businesses that exploit the communications revolution to get the best deal and price on goods and services almost anywhere on the globe. These organizations function as networks, with business functions accomplished by loosely aligned associations of independent producers, shippers, distributors, processors, marketers, financiers, and wholesalers. Such networked organizations pose special challenges to law enforcement and interdiction forces, because the very nature of a network is to be resistant to the disruption or

dismantling of individual business entities. As this strategy demonstrates, networked organizations are not immune from being attacked, disrupted, and dismantled. One way to severely disrupt a networked organization is to damage or destroy most of the elements in one horizontal layer of the network— especially a layer requiring critical contacts or skills—faster than the organization can replace them. For instance, typically, a Colombian trafficking organization may sell partially refined cocaine to a second organization, which routes it through final processing and then sells it to a broker. The broker may then sell to a second trafficking organization, which hires a transporter in conjunction with other traffickers to spread risk. The transporter typically moves the finished cocaine to Mexico in exchange for a portion of the profits. Once in Mexico, the cocaine is handled by entirely different sets of transporters and wholesalers. A Colombian transporter who can choose from among a dozen wholesalers cannot be disrupted simply by targeting a single wholesaler group. The transporter can, however, be significantly disrupted if, for example, eight of twelve wholesalers have been disrupted or taken out of operation. This Strategy describes how the U.S. Government, in concert with international allies, is seeking to target networks by attacking entire business sectors, such as the transporter sector. The strategy lays out several examples, including destroying the economic basis of the cocaine production business in South America by fumigating the coca crop, seizing enormous and unsustainable amounts of cocaine from transporters, and selectively targeting major organization heads for law enforcement action and, ultimately, extradition and prosecution in the United States.[17]

The supply reduction activities were basically the same in the Clinton administration. For example, the supply reduction goals in the 1998 NDCS were

1. eliminate illegal drug cultivation and production;

2. destroy drug-trafficking organizations;

3. interdict drug shipments;

4. encourage international cooperation; and

5. safeguard democracy and human rights.[18]

It is not surprising that the approach to supply reduction in the Clinton and Bush administrations is similar. Barry McCaffrey, the Drug Czar in the Clinton administration, was a military general with experience battling drug smugglers. John

Walters, the current director of ONDCP, had been a deputy director of ONDCP in charge of supply reduction. In fact, supply reduction initiatives started during the Clinton administration have been continued during the Bush administration. For example, Plan Colombia, an initiative started during the Clinton administration designed to reduce cocaine and heroin production in Colombia, was mentioned in Chapter 2. Plan Colombia has been expanded during the Bush administration.

How appropriate are activities such as Plan Colombia? In an editorial in the *Pittsburgh Post-Gazette* on May 2, 2005, the editorial writer stated:

> U.S. policy toward Colombia, America's third-largest aid beneficiary, has turned into a sinkhole of money and military resources over the past five years. The stated rationale for the heavy U.S. involvement in Colombia is the proposition that drug use in the United States can be reduced by suppression of production overseas. Colombia was the prime case in point for this approach. But it hasn't worked. Over five years, a U.S. financed air force, including helicopter gunships, has defoliated an estimated 1.3 million acres of coca plant and opium poppy fields in Colombia. In spite of this effort, the 90 percent of cocaine and 50 percent of the heroin on U.S. streets attributed to Colombian traffickers has not been reduced at all; it may even have increased. The price tag for "Plan Colombia," conceived in the Clinton years and carried out for the past four years under the Bush Administration, is nearly $3 billion. . . . Instead of pulling the plug on this unsuccessful enterprise, the Bush administration is now asking for $734 million more to finance it for yet another year. It is worth asking why.[19]

The supply reduction strategy is also failing in Mexico. In a 2005 article in the *Dallas Morning News*, the results of the U.S. approach are described:

> Mexico finally is fighting the war on drugs that the U.S. government has demanded for decades; a frontal assault on drug barons, their organizations and their merchandise, using the police and military in concert with U.S. intelligence. The results, Mexican and U.S. authorities say, have been impressive. Forty-six thousand people jailed on drug charges. President Vicente Fox said in a recent speech, 97 tons of cocaine seized, more than a million marijuana plants destroyed. It's been four years, Fox and U.S. officials said, of steady progress. But a rising chorus of voices in Mexico and the United States says the real results are record levels of violence, instability and corruption in Mexico, resurgent drug cartels, nearly 200 dead police officers and soldiers, along with millions of wasted dollars in a country where half the population of 105 million is poor . . . And the result in the United States?

No noticeable drop in the supply of cheap drugs—and an actual decline in the price of cocaine, according to a new U.N. report. Some analysts say Mexico's approach has not only failed to stanch the flow of drugs but also is destabilizing the young democracy ... Mexican criminal organizations dominate operations, controlling most of the thirteen primary drug distribution centers in the U.S. The violence of warring Mexican cartels has spilled over the border from Mexico to U.S. sites on the other side.[20]

Colombia and Mexico are not the only countries in which U.S. supply reduction activities have failed to achieve the desired objectives or have actually caused harm. In 2004, the Washington Office on Latin America, a think tank on Latin American human rights and social justice, published a study on the impact of U.S. drug policy on democracy in Latin America. The study found

... in one nation after another, U.S. drug control policies are undermining human rights and democracy and causing enormous damage to some of the most vulnerable populations in the hemisphere. The United States' insistence on zero tolerance for drug crops has led to massive forced eradication of coca and opium poppy crops, often the principal source of income for impoverished farmers. With few alternatives available, these families are ratcheted down into deeper poverty when their most important cash crop is destroyed. The region's militaries, which have not been held accountable for widespread human rights abuses and authoritarian dictatorships in the 1970s and 1980s, have been brought back into domestic law enforcement because the local police forces are either incapable or too corrupt to deal with the threat from drug trafficking and its associated violence.[21]

In the article from the *Dallas Morning News* regarding Mexico, there is a reference to a "new U.N. report." That is referring to the 2005 World Drug Report produced by the United Nations Office on Drugs and Crime.[22] This should be an objective analysis of the results of supply reduction activities, although it may be influenced by the predominance of the drug control approach of the United States on United Nations drug policies, as was discussed in Chapter 3. At the least, it is very unlikely that this U.N. report would be biased toward finding data that would prove that the United States supply reduction policies have failed, since that would be an indictment of U.N. policies as well. According to this report, worldwide opium production has been basically stable since the early 1990s. The production of cocaine had been decreasing until 2004, when the decreases in Colombia were offset by increases in the area under cultivation in Bolivia and Peru. According to the U.N. report, "This is a worrying loss of momentum for both countries, which had already made significant progress to curb coca production."[23] In spite of increased seizures of cocaine, "... prices dropped slightly in most of the major markets for the drug."[24] With regard to marijuana, "All indicators—production, seizures and consumption—suggest that the market at the global level is expanding further. For the time being, there is no reason to believe that this expansion will stop."[25]

Thus far, the information presented certainly indicates that the NDCS activities in the supply reduction area have failed and that some of the results have actually been harmful. Therefore, it is reasonable to conclude that at least some of the activities have been inappropriate. Specifically, crop eradication seems to hurt farmers in poor countries. The use of police and military to fight drug cartels has increased violence and instability in Latin America. In spite of the billions of dollars spent each year to reduce the supply of illegal drugs, neither the price, nor the purity, or availability of cocaine, heroin, marijuana, or methamphetamine has been impacted. Why?

Are the Supply Reduction Goals of the NDCS Impossible to Achieve?

Primarily, supply reduction goals cannot be achieved because of money. According to the U.N. report, the value of the global illegal drug market in 2003 was $13 billion at the production level, $94 billion at the wholesale level, and $322 billion at the retail level.[26] This is higher than the Gross Domestic Product (GDP) of 88 percent of the countries in the world.[27] That means there is a 623 percent markup from the production to the wholesale levels and a 243 percent increase from the wholesale to retail levels.

In 2003, the worldwide retail market value of marijuana products was $142 billion, cocaine was $71 billion, opiates (primarily heroin) was $65 billion, and methamphetamine, amphetamine, and ecstasy combined was $44 billion.[28] While the U.N. report does not give a breakdown of expenditures for illegal drugs by country, there are estimates by continent. North America spent $144 billion (retail) or 44 percent of the world's total on illegal drugs.[29] North America's share of cocaine expenditures was 62 percent; opiates, 14 percent; marijuana, 55 percent; and methamphetamine, amphetamine, and ecstasy, 57 percent.[30] Therefore, more than half of the world's retail expenditures on cocaine, marijuana, and stimulant drugs comes from North America.

At least with regard to cocaine and heroin, the vast majority of the money spent on these illegal drugs in the United States is by chronic users (those people with abuse or dependence disorders). According to a report prepared for ONDCP, 84.4 percent of the expenditures for cocaine were spent by chronic users of this drug and 94 percent of the money spent on heroin was by chronic users (these calculations were not reported for any other substances).[31]

Therefore, there are two huge forces that will maintain the supply of illegal drugs in this country regardless of efforts to control it: the tremendous money that is made from the wholesale and retail distribution of illegal drugs and the demand for illegal drugs created by chronic users. Let's discuss the money issue first.

Earlier in this chapter, the approaches from the 2005 NDCS that the United States has used to disrupt the profits in illegal drugs were described. If you will recall, the idea was to reduce the profitability of the illegal drug trade through escalating costs, diminishing profits, and unreliable suppliers. This was to be accomplished by fumigating coca, poppy, and marijuana crops, interdicting large quantities of illegal drugs from transporters, and arresting major cartel leaders. Clearly, none of this has worked. Let's analyze this a bit closer.

According to the U.N. report, opium poppy cultivation in 2004 in Afghanistan was higher than it has ever been[32] and the money generated by the heroin trade is 50 percent of that country's GDP.[33] In the report by the Washington Office on Latin America on the impact of U.S. drug policy in that region, the issue of crop eradication and alternative crop development programs is discussed:

> ... [there is] powerful evidence that forced coca eradication efforts are futile in the long run. In every case studied, short-term gains have been quickly reversed ... forced eradication efforts, and in particular aerial fumigation, often have dire consequences, generating social unrest, instability and violence ... Poverty, poor conditions for sustainable agricultural production, and the growing of crops for illicit drugs go hand-in-hand ... Increasingly, international donors are explicitly recognizing that simultaneous forced eradication and alternative development efforts are incompatible. The repressive nature of the former greatly limits, or hinders altogether, the cooperation needed for the later.[34]

> Two significant steps should be taken to reduce the harm caused by present drug control policies. First, cultivation of coca for traditional uses should not result in criminal sanctions. Second, coca and poppy production by small producers should be decriminalized; small growers should be considered "economic victims" with few viable options for survival, rather than criminals. This approach takes as its starting point the principle that all individuals have a right to life with dignity and hence should not be deprived of their only income source.[35]

Basically, coca plants and poppies are grown in very poor countries. The farmers who grow these products are doing so to support their families. When the United

States fumigates their crops, these farmers are naturally angry with us and unwilling to cooperate with alternative crop programs. As the situation in Afghanistan shows, as soon as these farmers were free of the control of the Taliban, they started growing poppies again. In Latin America, there will always be other farmers willing to grow coca and poppies when the land of current growers is fumigated. In other words, poor people will do whatever is necessary to make a living. This is not a moral issue for them. It is a subsistence issue.

There certainly could be debate about the economic necessity argument for those who grow marijuana domestically and for those people who produce methamphetamine. Given the fact that there are many alternatives to earn a livable wage in the United States, it can be assumed that enormous profits in illegal drugs is the primary motivation for those involved with growing marijuana and manufacturing methamphetamine in this country.

There are many levels between the growing of the plant (coca, poppy, marijuana) and the sale of illegal drugs on the street. The plants must be harvested, and the drugs must be produced, transported, distributed, and sold. A lot of workers are involved. The 2005 NDCS compared the illegal drug trade to any other business. So, like any other business, drug cartels are able to attract employees because they pay wages those workers cannot make in any other industry where they live. If you live in Bolivia and cannot find another job, you certainly would be happy to help make coca paste out of coca leaves (part of the process of turning coca leaves into cocaine).   ONGOING PROBLEM!

The point is that with the amounts of money and profit involved in the illegal drug trade, the United States can arrest the leaders of drug cartels but someone will replace them. We can destroy coca and poppy fields but someone else will grow them. We can stop a smuggling strategy but another one will be devised. We cannot stop poor people from doing what they need to do to survive and, as long as that survival involves working in the drug trade, there will never be a shortage of workers. We cannot stop people from wanting to control the illegal drug trade. Look at the economics of the situation. The United States is spending $7.7 billion this year to reduce the supply of illegal drugs. In North America alone, $144 billion a year is spent to purchase illegal drugs. It would be safe to conclude that those involved with the production and distribution of illegal drugs have more financial resources to find ways to get drugs into this country than the United States is willing to devote to the effort of stopping them. In short, if the demand for illegal drugs stays high, poverty and unemployment continue to be major problems in developing countries, and the profits in illegal drugs remain enormous, we will never stop the supply of illegal drugs.

So, what about reducing demand? In previous chapters, it has been pointed out that the prevention and treatment initiatives in the NDCS have not successfully reduced the demand for illegal drugs. In addition, the vast majority of cocaine and heroin is consumed by chronic users. Therefore, if demand is going to be impacted, the reduction has to come from chronic users. However, that reduction in demand will not come about through a constantly shifting focus on the drug "de jour."

At the beginning of this chapter, a *Newsweek* cover story on the methamphetamine "epidemic" was noted. Congress is now concerned about methamphetamine and wants to reduce the supply of this drug by controlling access to the precursor ingredients needed to manufacture it. A couple of years ago, there was a great deal of attention to the abuse of OxyContin, a prescription pain medication. Before that, ecstasy was in the news. Before that, there was a resurgence in the use of heroin. Then, there was the crack epidemic, the powder cocaine epidemic, etc. In each instance, the media had stories about people who become dependent on the current drug in vogue. But, as far as can be determined from the survey data that is available, there has not been any significant increase in the last 10 years in the overall percentage of Americans with drug dependence problems. Therefore, what apparently happens is that a certain proportion of individuals who are likely to become dependent on drugs use whatever is popular or available at the time and develop problems regardless of what that drug is. For example, if cocaine is too expensive, people who like stimulant drugs will use methamphetamine. People who use heroin will certainly use prescription pain medication if heroin is not available. That is not to say that methamphetamine or other specific drugs are not problems. They are. But, a problem like methamphetamine will not be stopped by trying to control the access to pseudoephedrine. If, by some miracle, people could be stopped from producing methamphetamine, the money to be made would motivate creative, criminal chemists to develop an alternative stimulant. The current strategy to reduce the supply of illegal drugs is analogous to plugging holes in a dyke, but every time a hole gets patched, another hole develops. The solution is to reduce demand by chronic users and implement effective methods to intervene in the evolution of new chronic users.

Conclusions

There is no part of the NDCS that illustrates its failure more clearly than supply reduction. Although more money is spent to reduce the supply of illegal drugs than is spent on any other part of the NDCS, there has been absolutely no impact on the price, purity, or availability of cocaine, heroin, marijuana, or methamphetamine during the 10-year time period discussed in this book. Not only has our approach failed to have the desired impact, there has also been harm created as a result of eradication, interdiction, and law enforcement efforts in foreign countries. The economics of this failure are easy to understand. The people of the United States spend nearly 20 times more on illegal drugs each year than the country spends trying to prevent these substances from reaching our streets. The production of illegal drugs such as cocaine and heroin occurs in poor countries of the world whose citizens rely on this industry for subsistence. Therefore, issues of poverty and unemployment in developing countries are major factors in the continuation of illegal drug production. The enormous profits involved ensures that there will always be people willing to run these businesses, workers to do the essential jobs, and creative energy to keep ahead of efforts to stop the activities. Furthermore, when the government focuses on reducing the supply of one illicit drug, the popularity of another drug increases. The solutions involve reducing the demand for illegal drugs by chronic drug users and preventing the development of new drug abusers. Without a focus on demand reduction, there is really no hope in reducing the supply of illicit drugs. These efforts not only waste money, they can cause damage to the most vulnerable participants in the production of illicit drugs and harm the reputation of the United States in other countries.

Nine

A New Model for a National Drug Control Policy

Introduction

The first two chapters of this book demonstrated that our NDCS over the past 10 years has failed in its major objectives. The supply of illegal drugs in the United States has not decreased. There have been no significant outcomes from prevention efforts. Treatment is the only area in which positive results have been demonstrated, and that is in spite of, rather than because of, the activities in our NDCS. After 10 years and nearly $145 billion, the lack of progress is inexcusable.

In Chapters 3–8, issues were discussed that are related to this failure. Some topics are banned from discussion among those involved in implementing the NDCS by federal officials (e.g., harm reduction, decriminalization, legalization) and, therefore, are not even allowed to be a part of a dialog on ways to improve the NDCS. On other topics (e.g., marijuana), there is such an inherent bias and knee-jerk reaction to suggestions on policy modifications that a reasonable discussion has never been possible. Some issues, such as effective strategies to reduce underage drinking, are opposed by the powerful alcohol lobby and, so, are not considered as essential parts of the NDCS. The futility of our supply reduction efforts is simply not acknowledged. The research that should guide prevention and treatment activities never seems to be able to significantly shift the emphasis in the demand reduction part of the NDCS.

The topics of Chapters 3–8 and the issues raised in these chapters were meant to stimulate a dialog that could result in a more effective NDCS through creative, innovative ideas. With this same objective, in this chapter, I will present my concept of a more effective NDCS. However, this is simply one version of what a NDCS could be. Hopefully, it will generate discussion and other ideas from the myriad of people with knowledge and experience in all parts of our NDCS. Only through an open and honest discussion without any taboo subjects will it be possible to make any progress on this enormous problem in our society.

Guiding Principles of a New NDCS

No More War

The tag line "War on Drugs" has to go. War has a military connotation and involves "good guys" and "bad guys." Is the war against drugs, drug users, drug sellers, drug manufacturers, or all of them? Who is the enemy? How do we know when we have won the war? If all of these questions seem ridiculous, they actually were the issues when the phrase "War on Drugs" was first used during the Reagan administration. The war was against drugs, drug users, drug sellers, and everyone else involved in production and distribution. The goal was a "drug-free" America and the weapons of the military and the criminal justice system were used in the battle to achieve this objective. Drug Czar Barry McCaffrey tried to tone down the rhetoric by saying that the effort was more like fighting cancer than fighting a war. However, the general public still sees the NDCS as a "war on drugs" and that contributes to stigma against addicts by creating a punishing rather than a helping mentality. Also, as has been shown in this book, it hasn't worked.

A Drug Is a Drug

The NDCS must deal with all mind-altering substances with addictive potential, including alcohol.[1] Because alcohol is a legal drug, the general public mistakenly believes that illicit drugs are more dangerous than alcohol. If the NDCS included alcohol, this misperception could be corrected. Furthermore, separating alcohol from illicit drugs is not just illogical; it also creates barriers in the development of effective prevention strategies. As was discussed in Chapters 5 and 6, prevention efforts have no hope of success unless the prevention and reduction of underage drinking are emphasized.

Addiction Is a Public Health Problem but Addicts Can Be Criminals

Alcohol and other drug addiction should be conceptualized as a public health problem and treated as such. Furthermore, those people who are addicted to alcohol and other drugs should not be seen as criminals *because of their addiction*. However, as was discussed in Chapter 7, there is a high percentage of people with antisocial personality disorder among the addicted population and many of these people commit criminal acts. Addicts should be treated compassionately and provided with appropriate care. Criminals who happen to have problems with alcohol or other drugs should be treated like criminals. Distinguishing who is who is very challenging. However, adopting an extreme position that addiction is always a public health problem or that all drug use is criminal behavior ignores the heterogeneity in the population of people called alcoholics or addicts.

Drug Use Is a Normal Part of Human Behavior, So the Goal Must Be to Reduce Harm

From the time that humans discovered they could achieve euphoria from ingesting mind-altering substances, they have engaged in this behavior. Throughout history, alcohol and other drug use can be found in nearly every society in all parts of the world. Since people cannot be stopped from engaging in this behavior, policies must be adopted to reduce the harm caused by alcohol and other drug use.

Alcohol and Other Drug Issues Do Not Exist in Isolation from Other Societal Problems

In Chapter 8, the fact that farmers in developing countries grow poppies and coca plants to earn a living was discussed. In Chapter 6, it was pointed out that the risk factors for substance abuse are the same as risk factors for other problems of young people and that many of these risk factors are related to poverty and family disintegration. In Chapter 7, research results were reported regarding the fact that addicts from low socioeconomic backgrounds are more likely to relapse. Therefore, while it is appealing to think about substance abuse problems as discreet issues that can be addressed through specific interventions, this is not an accurate reflection of reality. Certain aspects of supply and demand reduction may be impacted by the interventions that will be discussed in this chapter. However, the parts that are related to societal and global issues such as poverty and family breakdown must be part of larger efforts to address these problems.

Where Will the Money Come from to Implement These Recommendations?

Some of the recommendations in this chapter will cost money. It is best to discuss the issue of how to generate these resources prior to presenting the recommendations to avoid confounding the logic of the suggestions with the problem of paying for them. While there is a temptation to look at a reprioritization of the money that is already allocated to the NDCS, the danger in this approach is that the various interest groups involved with alcohol and other drug issues would be in a position of competing against each other. The goal of this book is to create an environment in which all of those groups are motivated to communicate about ways to create an effective NDCS. Competing for resources would be a barrier to achieving this goal.

A logical method to increase revenue to pay for these recommendations is through the federal excise tax on alcohol. In Chapter 5, the National Academy of Sciences report on underage drinking was discussed and this report included a recommendation on increasing federal excise taxes on alcohol as a method to reduce underage drinking. The current federal tax rates are $2.14 per 750 milliliter of 80 proof liquor, $0.33 per 6-pack of beer, and $0.21 per bottle of wine.[2] According to the National Academy of Sciences report

> By the standards of recent history, current tax rates are low ... Congress has not legislated increases in these taxes, so their real costs have been eroded by inflation. Restoring the federal excise tax on beer to its value in say, 1960, would require that it be increased by a factor of three ... Overall, alcoholic beverages are far cheaper today than they were in the 1960s and 1970s.[3]

Therefore, the federal excise tax could reasonably be doubled. Remember, this would only add $0.33 to a 6-pack of beer or about $0.05 a beer. In 2004, the federal excise tax on alcohol raised nearly $8 billion.[4] An increase of 100 percent in the excise tax should reduce consumption. Therefore, to be conservative about revenue, let's say that the increase in excise tax only increased the total amount collected by $6 billion. Therefore, there will be $6 billion a year to implement these recommendations.

This is not to suggest that I naively believe that Congress has the political courage to double the excise tax on alcohol. However, as the National Academy of Sciences report indicated, this increase would not even make beer as expensive as it was in 1960. So, it is a reasonable way to raise the money to support these recommendations.

Supply Reduction Recommendations

Supply reduction is an admittedly complex issue because it involves U.S. foreign relations policies, international treaties, the fight against terrorism, drug cartels, money laundering, and protection of our borders with Mexico and Canada. While all of these issues are important, concerns with foreign policy or homeland security must be separated from the focus here, which is the relationship between the supply of and demand for illicit drugs, because the priorities may be different. For example, the term narcoterrorism has been created by the government to connect the illegal drug trade to terrorism. In other words, the United States claims that terrorist organizations are involved in the illegal drug trade to support their activities. Perhaps this is true. However, the cocaine and heroin that enters the United States primarily comes from South America and Central America. This area of the world has a number of rebel organizations that may be battling their governments but it is really not a hotbed of terrorist activity directed at the United States, such as can be found in Southeast and Southwest Asia. In this regard, Afghanistan in Southwest Asia is producing a great deal of heroin but very little of this heroin enters the United States (most of it goes to Europe). Therefore, our interest in reducing heroin production in Afghanistan (described in Chapter 8) may have something to do with terrorist involvement in the drug trade but it is not about the supply of heroin in the United States. Since this is a book about drug policy rather than foreign policy or homeland security, the recommendations in this section only involve the relationship of supply reduction to demand reduction.

What is this relationship? Clearly, there has to be a demand for illicit drugs or there would be no market for them. As has been seen in this book, the demand for illicit drugs has been stable over time, with the only shifts being in the popularity of specific drugs at different times. If the demand for illicit drugs could be reduced somehow, the economics of supply and demand suggest that the supply would adjust without any intervention from government. On the other hand, if the federal government was able to significantly reduce the supply of some illegal drug but the demand remained stable, there would be a shift to whatever drug was available that produced a similar effect. For example, cocaine addicts would use methamphetamine if they couldn't get cocaine or if cocaine became outrageously expensive. And, remember from Chapter 8 that addicts consume the vast majority (nearly 85 percent) of the cocaine in this country. So, successful supply reduction activities are unlikely to have much impact on demand except to possibly shift the drugs people choose to use to get the effect they want. Because of this, supply reduction activities should be totally separated from demand reduction initiatives. In other words, the NDCS should only involve demand reduction and supply reduction should be the concern of some other government entity. This separation would remove supply reduction activities, which are primarily militaristic and law enforcement oriented, from any connection with demand reduction activities which should be primarily oriented to helping. Through this separation of function, the NDCS would be completely focused on the guiding principles discussed at the beginning of this section. In particular, there would not be any activities that perpetuate the analogy of a "war" on drugs.

However, I do want to discuss the viability of some of the supply reduction approaches because they clearly aren't working. First of all, the United States should stop crop eradication in developing countries. As was said in the previous chapter, crop eradication is an effort to disrupt the livelihood of poor people. It not only is ineffective; it alienates these farmers from the United States. It is difficult to believe that a Colombian farmer would resist growing an alternative crop if that farmer could make the same amount of money that is made growing coca. Therefore, this is an issue of global poverty and can only be solved by international efforts on that issue.

What about domestic crop eradication (i.e., destroying marijuana plants)? While these are not poor farmers growing pot plants to survive, the effort and expenditure of resources is not worth the result. Policies regarding marijuana will be discussed in this chapter but, for now, I believe that the resources devoted to finding and destroying marijuana plants could be better used in other areas. For example, methamphetamine labs are dangerous. There is a danger of explosion because of the volatility of the substances used and a risk of damage from the toxic chemicals produced during the manufacturing process. Needless to say, the drug that is produced is far more dangerous than marijuana as well. So, efforts aimed at locating and destroying marijuana plants would be better utilized in locating and destroying meth labs.

Some people argue that the legalization of drugs is the solution to the endless and seemingly impossible task of supply reduction. The reasoning is that, if currently illegal drugs were legal, the supply could be controlled. The production and distribution of drugs would become a legitimate business with government regulations and controls. If this argument is limited to heroin, cocaine, and methamphetamine for now, I believe that the legalization argument is a simplistic solution to a very complex issue. As was discussed in Chapter 3, the legalization of these illegal drugs has numerous complexities. It is naïve to believe that organizations involved with drug production and distribution will suddenly become respectable and ethical businesses if these drugs were legalized. In addition, the consequences of the use and abuse of cocaine, heroin, and methamphetamine cannot be ignored when discussing the legalization of these substances. The fact that these drugs are illegal and that access to them involves some risk does discourage some potential users. If these drugs were legal but extremely difficult to access, there would still be a black market. If they were legal but accessible, it would probably increase the number of users. Neither alternative is good.

Therefore, for the time being, agencies like the Coast Guard, Immigration and Customs Enforcement, Customs and Border Protection, and the DEA should be allowed to continue efforts to interdict heroin, cocaine, and methamphetamine so there is at least some management of the quantities of these drugs that get into the country. If these efforts were largely confined to smuggling, large-scale marketers, and meth labs, they wouldn't help much in reducing the supply of drugs but they wouldn't be hurting the most vulnerable participants in the illicit drug trade either. In addition, there are practical advantages beyond drug inter-diction for these agencies to be involved in this effort. For example, it provides an opportunity for the personnel of these agencies to engage in operational field work and technological advances can be tested in real situations.

In the current NDCS, supply reduction also includes domestic law enforcement activities directed against drug users and against small-scale drug distributors who sell drugs to support their own addiction. I do not consider these activities supply reduction since the focus of these efforts is on drug users. Therefore, these issues will be discussed in a later section of this chapter.

The New NDCS

In this new approach to a NDCS, the term "demand reduction" would not be used because many of the strategies are designed to manage, rather than reduce, demand. There would be three broad areas of emphasis: prevention of addictive disorders, harm management, and treatment. Each of these will be discussed in detail.

Prevention of Addictive Disorders

The overall goal of the activities in this area is to reduce the number of people with substance abuse or substance dependence disorders. This means that there would be a heavy emphasis on young people, but there would also be a focus on people who are using alcohol and other drugs but who have not developed an abuse or dependence disorder.

Before describing the activities included in this area, let me explain what is *not* included. In Chapter 6, the risk and protective factor theory of prevention was discussed. It was pointed out that many of the risk factors for substance abuse in-volved poverty, community dysfunction, and family disintegration. Furthermore, the risk factors for substance abuse are the same as the risk factors for other youth problems such as violence, delinquency, teen pregnancy, and dropping out of school. Therefore, it does not make sense to separate substance abuse prevention efforts that are designed to reduce these risk factors from the broader societal issues related to poverty, community dysfunction, and family disintegration. In fact, it may be counterproductive to design interventions to reduce these risk factors and to call them "substance abuse prevention" since it can isolate these programs from broader community efforts. This is not to say that efforts to reduce these risk factors should be eliminated. On the contrary, there should be more intensive, evidence-based, comprehensive efforts at all levels designed to reduce risk factors for the development of these problems. However, these initiatives should not be called "substance abuse prevention."

The primary approach to preventing the development of addictive disorders in young people would be through the implementation of policies, laws, and regulations designed to impact young people's access to and use of alcohol. As was discussed in Chapters 5 and 6, underage drinking is the primary drug abuse problem among minors, and young people who use alcohol are far more likely to use illicit drugs than those young people who do not use these substances. Since research has already demonstrated the effectiveness of strategies to reduce smoking and underage drinking such as increases in excise taxes, restrictions on retail outlets, "sting operations," "zero tolerance" of underage drinking, and keg registration, these approaches should be standardized across states and local communities. In addition, the recommendations of the National Academy of Sciences with regard to underage drinking (described in Chapter 5) should be implemented. However, the recommendations with regard to marketing of alcohol should be broadened. As was discussed in Chapter 6, one lesson from the effectiveness of efforts to reduce youth smoking was that a public awareness campaign can be successful if it is combined with restrictions on the marketing of tobacco. The same strategy should be applied to alcohol. Therefore, the content of alcohol advertising should be limited to product attributes. While many people find alcohol advertising to be creative, amusing, and provocative, it is clearly designed to encourage underage and excessive drinking.

The standard argument used by the alcohol industry is that such restrictions are a violation of first amendment protections of freedom of expression. First of all, there are all sorts of restrictions on the content of what can be shown on television. Certain four letter words are censored and frontal nudity or sexual acts are not shown on network television. However, the issue of protection of expression can be entirely avoided if the alcohol industry would voluntarily agree to marketing restrictions. While this may sound inconceivable, the tobacco industry agreed to restrictions to avoid other consequences, such as additional legislative actions controlling their marketing. There are many legislative acts that would have a detrimental effect on alcohol sales and distribution including a further lowering of the minimum blood alcohol content for DUI and regulation of alcohol by the Food and Drug Administration. If elected officials had the political courage, the alcohol industry could be pressured to accept marketing restrictions by the threat of legislative actions that would lower profits even further than what would result from advertising restrictions.

If there were restrictions on alcohol marketing and if access to alcohol was more difficult for minors, then a concentrated public awareness campaign regarding tobacco, alcohol, and illicit drug use would have more likelihood of impacting the use patterns of young people. Therefore, the new NDCS would include a "media campaign" developed along the same lines as the "truth" campaign designed by the American Legacy Foundation (described in Chapter 6).

The prevention of addictive disorders also would include interventions designed to decrease the probability of those who already use alcohol and other drugs to develop abuse or dependence disorders. There is strong research evidence that brief interventions, often delivered by physicians or other healthcare providers, are extremely effective in moderating the drinking patterns of heavy alcohol users who have not developed an alcohol use disorder.[5] Screening to determine the alcohol and other drug use of patients can be accomplished through responses to short questionnaires developed for this purpose. The types of questions on screening instruments are very similar to other health-related questions that people are accustomed to completing in medical facilities prior to appointments. If this screening and brief intervention process were a routine part of primary care and emergency room procedures, it could be very effective in intervening with problem drinkers and drug users before dependence develops. An added benefit would be in the identification and referral of people with substance abuse disorders whose utilization of the healthcare system is related to their untreated alcohol and other drug problem, costing nearly $63 billion a year (see Table 1.2). If you recall from Chapter 7, there are about 19 million Americans with substance use disorders who do not believe they need treatment. By identifying some of these people through screening in healthcare settings, more of them might be willing to access treatment services.

Harm Management

This area would be the core of a new NDCS. Acknowledging and accepting that alcohol and other drug use and abuse has always been and will always be a reality allows us to develop strategies to reduce the enormous human and economic harm that results from substance abuse. First, let's discuss harm management strategies regarding alcohol. In the prevention of addictive disorders section, policies, laws, and regulations were mentioned to reduce underage drinking. Many of these strategies can also reduce the harm of alcohol abuse. For example, increasing excise taxes has been shown to reduce the consequences of alcohol abuse among adults as well as underage drinkers. Mandatory training for servers of alcohol can help prevent them from providing alcohol to inebriated customers. Sobriety checkpoints reduce the incidence of DUIs. However, it is important to identify effective policies, laws, and regulations and create the motivation for uniformity across jurisdictions. The federal government did this with regard to blood alcohol levels for DUI and could do so in other areas. This would help to alleviate the pressure of special interest lobbying on state and local officials. For example, in Nevada, the state I live in, the effort to lower the blood alcohol level from 0.10 to 0.08 for DUIs was consistently defeated because of pressure from the casino and alcohol industries. However, the federal mandate for states to lower the blood alcohol level or risk the loss of highway funds was effective in overcoming this special interest lobbying. However, more needs to be done in certain areas to manage the harm caused by alcohol abuse. For example, in all states, the consequences for DUIs should include an assessment to determine if the individual has an alcohol abuse or dependence disorder. Since approximately one-third of drivers arrested or convicted of a DUI each year are repeat offenders[6] (and thus are likely to have an alcohol use disorder), this assessment is crucial. Persons convicted of a DUI should have an ignition interlock installed in their cars. These devices are breathalyzers that will not allow the car to start until a breath sample is given that has a lower blood alcohol content than the device has programmed into it. First-time offenders could have the device removed after a year of no further offenses. Second-time offenders would have the devices permanently. Obviously, someone can disable the device or circumvent the system in other ways. However, these are harm management procedures. There is no way to implement a foolproof system in a democratic society.

Additionally, bars and restaurants that serve alcohol should have breathalyzers for customers to use before they leave the premises. Customers with blood alcohol content of 0.08 or above should be assisted with transportation. If a customer with a high blood alcohol content refused alternative transportation, the business should be required to notify the police or face a suspension of their liquor license. Customers who are clearly inebriated and refuse to take a breathalyzer should also be reported.

If this seems like an onerous burden on businesses that serve alcohol, you probably would not feel that way if someone you loved was killed by a drunk driver leaving a bar. Theoretically, it is the drinker who should be responsible enough to arrange for a safe way to get home if he or she intends to drink. However, alcohol impairs judgment. So drinkers cannot be relied upon to make good decisions. Therefore, the establishment that is making a profit on excessive alcohol use will have to be inconvenienced to reduce the harm that drunk drivers cause.

In Chapter 3, a variety of harm reduction approaches regarding illicit drug use were discussed. One of the most sensible, which has been adopted in cities in the

United States in spite of government opposition, is needle exchange programs. Needle exchanges, where intravenous drug users can exchange a used syringe for a sterile one, should be available in all locations where there is widespread injection of drugs.

In addition, drug consumption facilities (see Chapter 3) should be developed. These facilities would be secure, supervised clinics where illicit drugs could be used by chronic addicts. Since this is such a controversial and radical move for the United States, this should be done on a small scale in receptive communities and thoroughly evaluated to determine the impact on drug use and the consequences of drug abuse, such as crime and infectious diseases. There would need to be a process to assess potential clients to determine the chronicity of addiction, other physical and mental health conditions, and to assess the viability of treatment as an alternative to continued drug use. Those clients with infectious diseases would have to agree to treatment or management of these conditions. As in Europe, consumption rooms should offer a range of social and health services for chronic addicts.

There is a question of what drugs should be allowed to be used in such a facility. Heroin is an obvious choice since a major purpose of drug consumption rooms is to create a safe environment to inject drugs. Furthermore, people intoxicated with heroin are generally not unruly so disruptive behavior should not be a frequent problem among heroin addicts. However, should cocaine or methamphetamine be allowed? These stimulant drugs can result in violent or paranoid behavior. What about alcohol consumption rooms for chronic alcoholics? Should only drug injection be allowed or could snorting or smoking be conducted in a drug consumption room? The most cautious way to proceed would be to initially restrict consumption rooms for chronic, injecting heroin users. If this approach is successful, it could be expanded to include other drugs and other methods of use. For example, it might be viable to have residential consumption facilities for chronic alcoholics or cocaine addicts where the results of their drug ingestion can be monitored and managed. The concept is to try some novel methods to manage the harm from chronic drug addiction and to expand those methods that produce results.

An issue related to drug consumption rooms is the source of the drugs that are consumed. In the European model of consumption rooms, the clients supply the drugs. Of course, this can cause problems since the purity of the drugs and the substances used as adulterants would be unknown. To combat this problem, law enforcement agencies that acquire supplies of illegal drugs from arrests could provide the drugs in drug consumption rooms (after assessing the content of the substances) and eliminate any problems with contaminates and overdoses. In addition, this procedure would be an ideal way to assess the impact of reduced demand for illegal drugs on the supply in a community. For example, let's say there was a drug consumption facility in Seattle for chronic heroin addicts. Heroin is supplied in the facility. So the addicts are not purchasing the drug on the streets. Since chronic addicts consume most of the heroin, this would reduce the demand for heroin in Seattle. Chronic addicts would not have to raise money to buy drugs through illegal activities or panhandling and the market for drug traffickers would be significantly reduced. The ironic aspect of this scenario is that the way to impact the supply of illegal drugs (and the profit of drug traffickers) might be to reduce the street demand for illegal drugs by chronic addicts by providing them with interdicted drugs. Again, remember that the goal is to manage the harm from drug abuse. If chronic addicts, who are going to continue to use drugs no matter what, have a regulated supply and do not have to get money to purchase drugs, many potential sources of harm will be reduced.

It should be pointed out that consumption rooms are not a substitute for abstinence-based treatment or opiate substitution therapy such as methadone or buprenorphine. As will be discussed in the next section, these treatment options should be readily available and easily accessed by addicts. In addition, traditional treatment and opiate substitution therapies should be the first alternatives for injecting drug addicts. However, as was shown in Table 7.1, the drop out rate for clients in methadone treatment was much higher than in any other form of treatment. Therefore, the development of drug consumption rooms acknowledges the reality that many addicts will continue to use drugs in spite of numerous treatment episodes and involvement in a variety of treatment alternatives. In addition, some addicts will refuse treatment. In the new NDCS, the goal is to reduce the harm that these individuals cause themselves and society. Drug consumption rooms will contribute to achieving this goal.

Managing the harm of drug abuse also requires rethinking how drug possession is handled. If drug abuse is a public health issue, it would not seem logical to arrest people for drug possession. However, it is also important to encourage and motivate drug abusers to get treatment and the criminal justice system can be used for this purpose. A possible solution that does not involve the arrest process but doesn't eliminate the coercive power of the criminal justice system is to treat drug possession as a misdemeanor. A citation would be issued but the fine would be waived if the offender completed a drug and mental health assessment and agreed to follow the recommendations. Assessment centers would have to be conveniently located for users. Repeated citations would result in a drug court referral. The only scenario in which someone would be incarcerated for drug possession would be if the individual continually refused to complete an assessment and would not either enter treatment or use drugs safely in a drug consumption facility. Obviously, a drug user with a serious mental health problem (e.g., schizophrenia) should not be incarcerated for an extended length of time. The only purpose of incarceration would be to force the individual to complete an assessment.

Small-scale drug distributors, who sell drugs to support their addiction, should be arrested and referred to drug court. However, a drug consumption facility should be one alternative if the person is appropriate for that approach.

Finally, how should harm be managed with regard to marijuana? Clearly, there is a need for policy modifications. However, there is insufficient information to warrant complete legalization of marijuana. Therefore, the following is recommended:

1. The Controlled Substances Act should be revised and marijuana should be reclassified from its current Schedule I classification.

2. Personal use at home should be decriminalized.

3. The cultivation of a small number of marijuana plants on a person's property should be decriminalized.

4. Different decriminalization and legalization schemes should be implemented in confined locations such as cities or counties so each policy modification can be thoroughly evaluated.

5. The recommendation from the Institute of Medicine's report regarding the use of marijuana for people suffering from certain chronic conditions should be adopted (see Chapter 4) and state medical marijuana laws should be supported by the federal government.

6. The federal government should support, encourage, and allow research on marijuana using plants with THC content similar to what is sold on the street.

7. Large-scale distribution should continue to be a criminal offense.

Treatment

As was discussed in Chapter 7, public-sector treatment could be improved in several ways. First, there must be enough treatment facilities and treatment availability so that anyone who needs and wants treatment can get it. Second, the length of treatment should be at least 90 days as recommended by the National Institute on Drug Abuse. Third, there must be a variety of treatment settings and treatment alternatives available in order to meet the needs of the addicted population. For example, more short-term and long-term residential treatment programs should be developed. Opiate substitution therapies (i.e., methadone and buprenorphine) must be easily accessed by those heroin addicts who are appropriate and interested in this type of treatment. Fourth, there must be some kind of continuing care or support for those addicts who fit the chronic medical condition concept of addiction. Fifth, treatment programs must be able to provide care for co-occurring mental disorders and support services for other client needs.

This vision of the treatment system in a new NDCS involves multiservice treatment facilities that can provide for the diverse needs of the public-sector treatment population. This means that a variety of levels of service would be available (long- and short-term residential, outpatient, and intensive outpatient), a multidisciplinary professional staff (e.g., addiction counselors, medical personnel, mental health professionals) would be provided, and a seamless method to provide ancillary services such as vocational training, financial management, and self-care skills would be in place. Services such as child care would be provided to remove barriers to treatment. There must be provisions for regular follow-up contact with treatment professionals and/or attendance at some kind of support group. All of this requires an infusion of resources to upgrade the public-sector treatment system.

One of the guiding principles in the beginning of this chapter was that addiction is a public health problem but addicts can be criminals. In the framework of conceptualizing addiction as a public health problem, everything should be done to provide appropriate treatment for anyone who needs it and wants it. Furthermore, every effort should be made to manage the harm that is caused by this public health problem. The discussion so far has dealt with both of these issues. However, the issue of the criminal addict also must be considered. When the term "criminal addict" is used, this does not include those who are arrested for possession of illegal drugs, for selling drugs to support an addiction, or for public intoxication. The harm management section dealt with these problems.

In Chapter 7, the large percentage of public-sector clients with antisocial personality disorder was discussed. Also, it was noted that over one-third of referrals to public-sector treatment came from the criminal justice system. If you read the criteria for antisocial personality disorder again in Chapter 7, it is reasonable to assume that many of these criminal justice referrals have this condition. Unfortunately, it is not easy to diagnose antisocial personality disorder, especially among individuals with addiction problems because many addicts commit criminal acts. They may commit these acts in order to get money to support their addiction or they may act criminally as a result of the effect of alcohol and other drugs. To really determine which client has antisocial personality disorder and which client's primary problem is an addictive disorder, you have to wait and see what happens when the client has been clean and sober for an extended period of time. The client with antisocial personality disorder will continue to behave inappropriately and/or criminally.

However, as has been discussed previously, many or most clients relapse. So, if clients don't stay sober long enough, how can you tell who has antisocial personality disorder and who doesn't? The fact is, it probably doesn't matter. If someone commits a criminal act, the person has to have consequences for that behavior regardless of what their problem is. So, there should be sufficient treatment available in state and federal correctional institutions to serve inmates with addictive disorders. Additionally, the incarceration period provides an opportunity to assess inmates for other mental disorders since, theoretically, they should not be using alcohol or other drugs while in prison. Along with treatment services in prison, inmates must be able to access professional and support group services after their release to increase their chances of remaining sober.

Some people with addictive disorders who are incarcerated for crimes and treated while in prison may clearly be candidates for harm management strategies such as consumption rooms. It may be clear to treatment personnel that relapse is very likely or the client may have been unsuccessful with postincarceration sobriety on more than one occasion. In these cases, the consumption room should be an option and residential consumption rooms might be the most effective way to manage harm for postincarcerated, relapsing clients.

If, in spite of treatment and/or consumption rooms, the individual continues to commit crimes, there is a high probability that the individual has antisocial personality disorder. Further treatment is a waste of resources in these cases. When the individual is not incarcerated, he or she should be strongly encouraged to use consumption rooms and maintain a crime-free lifestyle. Otherwise, there will be forced sobriety during incarceration. For some antisocial personality disordered clients, this clear choice, with one option allowing the continued use of alcohol and other drugs and the other option forced abstinence, will be sufficient to modify behavior.

Conclusions

At the beginning of this book, I told you that I consider myself an insider on the so-called "War on Drugs." For the past 12 years, I have worked on federal projects designed to help with the demand reduction side of the NDCS. For the most part, the people I have encountered that are doing this same kind of work are dedicated, committed, hardworking professionals whose primary goal is to help those with addictive disorders or prevent young people from developing these conditions. Many of the lower-level federal bureaucrats are also sincere people trying their best to manage a complex system. When we all get together at meetings, the failure of the NDCS is like the elephant in the living room. Some people may talk about it in small informal groups outside of the meetings. Most people pretend that it is not there and focus their time on trivial issues that create a false sense that important issues are being dealt with. However, everyone always seems frustrated with the lack of progress. There may be numerous opinions about why we can't make more headway but everyone I know at this level of government and project management acknowledges that we aren't. Clearly, a totally new approach is needed.

This framework for a new NDCS is only one model from an infinite number of possibilities. Some of the concepts and recommendations presented in this chapter may make you uncomfortable or irritated. For example, the idea of drug consumption rooms can elicit strong negative reactions. If you drink, you might not like the idea of increased alcohol excise taxes or restrictions on retail outlets. However, I believe that, no matter what parts of this new model you find useful and what parts you find ridiculous, there are two irrefutable facts that require consideration of a radically new NDCS: (1) The guiding principles of our current NDCS are untenable and (2) The strategies that have been developed on the basis of these principles have failed. If there is agreement on these facts, then there can be an open, honest, and creative dialog to develop a workable NDCS that has the potential to reduce the harm caused by alcohol and other drugs. However, without acknowledgment of these facts, the government officials who create the NDCS will continue to pursue strategies, activities, and initiatives that increase the problem they are trying to solve.

Notes

Chapter 1

1. Office of National Drug Control Policy, 2004. The price and purity of illicit drugs: 1981 through the second quarter of 2003. http://www.whitehousedrugpolicy.gov/publications/price_purity/.

2. Terminology can be challenging in this field. In this book, the term "illegal" will be used to refer to drugs that are unlawful to possess and use under most circumstances (e.g., marijuana, heroin, cocaine, methamphetamine, ecstasy, LSD). The term "illicit" will be used to refer to illegal drugs and those substances that are legal to possess in many cases but can be used illegally (e.g., prescription pain medications, inhalants). Addiction can refer to a dependence on alcohol or illicit drugs. Since many people associate "addiction" with illicit drugs and "alcoholism" with alcohol, both terms will frequently be used in this book. However, whenever the term "addiction" is used, understand that it can refer to dependence on alcohol and/or illicit drugs. Similarly, alcohol is a drug. Therefore, any discussion of "drugs" includes alcohol. However, since many people distinguish alcohol from illicit drugs, the term "alcohol and other drugs" will be used to avoid any confusion. If the discussion is only about drugs other than alcohol, the term "illicit drugs" will help readers understand that alcohol is not a part of the discussion. Finally, "substance abuse" and "substance dependence" are terms used for conditions that are diagnosed based on the *Diagnostic and statistical manual of mental disorders*, the "bible" used by psychiatrists, psychologists, and other mental health professionals. These conditions can refer to alcohol or illicit drugs. "Abuse" is less severe than "dependence" but either condition requires some type of treatment.

3. Office of National Drug Control Policy, 2005. The President's national drug control strategy. Chapter III. Disrupting the market: Attacking the economic basis of the drug trade. http://www.whitehousedrugpolicy.gov/publications/policy/ndcs05/.39.

4. Data from this survey is not available prior to 1991.

5. L. D. Johnston, P. M. O'Malley, J. G. Bachman, and J. E. Schulenberg, 2006. *Monitoring the future national results on adolescent drug use: Overview of key findings, 2005.* NIH Publication No. 06-5882. Bethesda, MD: National Institute on Drug Abuse.

6. Since I know of instances in which federal funding was cut from those who criticized federal policies, I asked to be reassigned from my responsibilities as director of my center prior to the publication of this book. In that way, the programs in the center would be protected from any association with the opinions in this book.

7. The National Youth Anti-Drug Media Campaign includes, among other things, commercials on television designed to influence young people to stay away from illicit drugs.

8. Public Broadcasting System, 2000. Thirty years of America's drug war: A chronology. http://www.pbs.org/wgbh/pages/frontline/shows/drugs/cron/.

9. A. Allen. 2000. Portrait of a drug czar. Salon.com. http://dir.salon.com/health/feature/2000/08/30/czar/index.html.

10. Ibid.

11. Office of National Drug Control Policy, 2006. National Drug Control Strategy FY 2007 Budget Summary: February 2006. http://www.whitehousedrugpolicy.gov/publications/policy/07budget/.

12. Office of National Drug Control Policy, 2004. The economic costs of drug abuse in the United States 1992–2002. http://www.whitehousedrugpolicy.gov/publications/economic_costs/.

13. Ibid.

14. H. Harwood, 2000. Updating estimates of the economic costs of alcohol abuse in the United States: Estimates, update, methods, and data. National Institute on Alcohol Abuse and Alcoholism. http://pubs.niaaa.nih.gov/publications/economic-2000/alcoholcost.PDF.

15. Office of National Drug Control Policy, 2004. The economic costs of drug abuse in the United States 1992–2002. http://www.whitehousedrugpolicy.gov/publications/economic_costs/.

16. National Institute on Alcohol Abuse and Alcoholism, 1996. State trends in alcohol problems: 1979–92. http://pubs.niaaa.nih.gov/publications/alcdth96.pdf.

Chapter 2

1. Office of National Drug Control Policy, 1996. The national drug control strategy: 1996. http://www.ncjrs.org/pdffiles/strat96.pdf.

2. Office of National Drug Control Policy, 2005. The President's national drug control strategy: February 2005. Appendix A: National drug control budget summary. http://www.whitehousedrugpolicy.gov/publications/policy/ndcs05/.

3. Ibid., 10.

4. Ibid., 11.

5. Office of National Drug Control Policy, 1996. The national drug control strategy: 1996. http://www.ncjrs.org/pdffiles/strat96.pdf.

6. Office of National Drug Control Policy, 1997. The national drug control strategy: 1997. http://www.ncjrs.org/htm/toc.htm.

7. Office of National Drug Control Policy, 1998. The national drug control strategy: 1998. http://www.ncjrs.org/ondcppubs/publications/pdf/budget98.pdf.

8. Office of National Drug Control Policy, 1999. The national drug control strategy: 1999. http://www.ncjrs.org/ondcppubs/publications/policy/99ndcs/99ndcs.pdf.

9. Office of National Drug Control Policy, 2000. The national drug control strategy: 2000. http://www.ncjrs.org/ondcppubs/publications/policy/ndcs00/strategy2000.pdf.

10. John Mintz, 2005. Probe faults system for monitoring U.S. borders. *The Washington Post*, April 11. http://www.washingtonpost.com/wp- dyn/content/article/2005/04/10/AR2005041001382.html (accessed August 18, 2005).

11. Office of National Drug Control Policy, 2002. The President's national drug control strategy: February 2002. http://www.whitehousedrugpolicy.gov/publications/policy/ndcs02/.

12. Office of National Drug Control Policy, 2003. The President's national drug control strategy: February 2003. http://www.whitehousedrugpolicy.gov/publications/policy/ndcs03/index.html.

13. Ibid., 26.

14. Office of National Drug Control Policy, 2004. The President's national drug control strategy: March 2004. http://www.whitehousedrugpolicy.gov/publications/policy/ndcs04/index.h tml.

15. Office of National Drug Control Policy. 2005. The President's national drug control strategy: February 2005. Appendix A: National drug control budget summary. http://www.whitehousedrugpolicy.gov/publications/policy/ndcs05/.

16. Office of National Drug Control Policy. 1999. The national drug control strategy: 1999.http://www.ncjrs.org/pdffiles/strat99.pdf.

17. Ibid.

18. Ibid.

19. Office of National Drug Control Policy, 2002. The President's national drug control strategy: February 2002. http://www.whitehousedrugpolicy.gov/publications/policy/ndcs02/.

20. Hereafter, this survey will be referred to as the National Household Survey. The name was changed in 2002 from the National Household Survey on Drug Abuse to the National Household Survey on Drug Use and Health. The term "National Household Survey" will be used to discuss all editions of this survey.

21. The Monitoring the Future Survey has more 8th graders than 10th graders and more 10th graders than 12th graders in its sample. However, a weighted average, based on sample size, would bias the average toward the younger students. In the most recent National Household Survey, a comparison between the results of the

Monitoring the Future Survey and the National Household Survey was conducted using a simple average computation of the combined 8th, 10th, and 12th grade results from the Monitoring the Future Survey. Therefore, a simple average computation was used here.

22. The differences between the results of the Monitoring the Future Survey and the National Household Survey may be a reflection of the different survey methods employed. Therefore, it is more important to compare changes over time within a survey rather than results between surveys.

23. Office of Applied Studies, Substance Abuse and Mental Health Services Administration, 2003. National Survey on Drug Use and Health. Chapter 8: Substance dependence, abuse, and treatment. http://oas.samhsa.gov/nhsda/2k2nsduh/2k2SoFw.pdf.

24. Center for Disease Control, 2005. Youth risk behavior surveillance survey. http://www.cdc.gov/healthyyouth/yrbs/about_yrbss.htm.

25. Center for Disease Control, 2006. Youth risk behavior surveillance—United States, 2005. *Morbidity and mortality weekly report*, June 9. http://www.cdc.gov/mmwr/PDF/SS/SS5505.pdf .

26. Office of Applied Studies, Substance Abuse and Mental Health Services Administration, 2005. Results from the 2004 National Survey on Drug Use and Health: National findings. Chapter 5: Initiation of substance use. http://oas.samhsa.gov/nsduh/2k4nsduh/ 2k4Results/2k4Results.htm#ch5.

27. Office of National Drug Control Policy, 1999. The national drug control strategy: 1999. http://www.ncjrs.org/pdffiles/strat99.pd.45.

28. Office of Applied Studies, Substance Abuse and Mental Health Services Administration, Office of Applied Studies, 2004. National Household Survey on Drug Abuse: Substance dependence, abuse, and treatment tables—Tables H.57 to H.70. http://oas.samhsa.gov/NHSDA/2k1NHSDA/vol2/appendixh_5.htm#tableh.58.

29. Office of Applied Studies, Substance Abuse and Mental Health Services Administration, 2005. National Household Survey on Drug Use and Health, Appendix H: Selected prevalence tables—Table H.38. http://oas.samhsa.gov/nsduh/2k4nsduh/2k4Results/appH.htm#tabh.38.

30. Office of National Drug Control Policy, 1999. The national drug control strategy: 1999. http://www.ncjrs.org/pdffiles/strat99.pdf.

31. Office of National Drug Control Policy, 2004. The President's national drug control strategy: Data supplement. http://www.whitehousedrugpolicy.gov/publications/policy/ndcs04/data_suppl.htm.35.

32. Office of National Drug Control Policy, 1999. The national drug control strategy: 1999. http://www.ncjrs.org/pdffiles/strat99.pd.45.

33. United States Department of Justice, National Drug Intelligence Center, 2005. National threat assessments: National drug threat assessment. http://www.usdoj.gov/ndic/topics/ndtas.htm (accessed August 10, 2005).

34. Ibid., 2001 report, 9.

35. Ibid., 2002 report, v.

36. Ibid., 2003 report, v.

37. Ibid., 2004 report, vi.
38. Ibid., 2005 report, vi.
39. Ibid., 2001 report, 10.
40. Ibid., 2002 report, vi.
41. Ibid., 2003 report, vi.
42. Ibid., 2004 report, vi.
43. Ibid., 2005 report, vi.
44. Ibid., 2001 report, 21.
45. Ibid., 2002 report, vi.
46. Ibid., 2003 report, vi.
47. Ibid., 2004 report, vii.
48. Ibid., 2005 report, vii.
49. Ibid., 2001 report, 42–43.
50. Ibid., 2002 report, vii.
51. Ibid., 2003 report, vi.
52. Ibid., 2004 report, vi.
53. Ibid., 2005 report, vi.
54. Office of National Drug Control Policy, 2004. The President's national drug control strategy: Data supplement. http://www.whitehousedrugpolicy.gov/publications/policy/ndcs04/data_suppl.htm.47.
55. Ibid., 49.
56. Office of National Drug Control Policy, 2004. The economic costs of drug abuse in the United States 1992–2002. http://www.whitehousedrugpolicy.gov/publications/economic_costs/.
57. National Institute of Justice, Arrestee Drug Abuse Monitoring Program, No date. 1997 annual report on adult and juvenile arrestees. http://www.ncjrs.org/nij/textrev.pdf_4.
58. National Institute of Justice, Arrestee Drug Abuse Monitoring Program, No date. Drug and alcohol use and related matters among arrestees 2003. http://www.ojp.usdoj.gov/nij/adam/ADAM2003.pdf.
59. Office of National Drug Control Policy, 2004. The economic costs of drug abuse in the United States 1992–2002. http://www.whitehousedrugpolicy.gov/publications/economic_costs/.
60. Office of National Drug Control Policy, 2004. The President's national drug control strategy: Data supplement. http://www.whitehousedrugpolicy.gov/publications/policy/ndcs04/data_su ppl.htm. 41.
61. Ibid., 42.
62. Ibid., 44.
63. Ibid., 43.
64. Ibid., 46.
65. Center for Disease Control, 2006. Youth risk behavior surveillance—United States, 2005. *Morbidity and mortality weekly report*, June 9. http://www.cdc.gov/mmwr/PDF/SS/SS5505.pdf.

66. G. L. Fisher and T. C. Harrison, 2005. *Substance abuse: Information for school counselors, social workers, therapists, and counselors.* 3rd ed. Boston: Pearson.

67. U.S. Department of Education, National Center for Education Statistics, 2005. *The condition of education 2005.* NCES 2005-094. Washington, D.C.: U.S. Government Printing Office.

68. Parents' Resource Institute for Drug Education, 2005. PRIDE questionnaire report for grades 6 thru 12, 2003–2004 PRIDE national summary/ Grades 6 thru 12. http://www.pridesurveys.com/ (accessed August 11, 2005).

69. Office of National Drug Control Policy, 2004. The economic costs of drug abuse in the United States 1992–2002. http://www.whitehousedrugpolicy.gov/publications/economic_costs/.

70. Office of National Drug Control Policy, 2004. The President's national drug control strategy: Data supplement, p. 47. http://www.whitehousedrugpolicy.gov/publications/policy/ndcs04/data_suppl.htm.

71. Ibid., 49.

72. Ibid.

73. National Institute of Justice, Arrestee Drug Abuse Monitoring Program, No date. 1998 annual report on drug use among adult and juvenile arrestees. http://www.ncjrs.org/pdffiles/175656.pdf.

74. National Institute of Justice, Arrestee Drug Abuse Monitoring Program, No date. Drug and alcohol use and related matters among arrestees 2003. http://www.ojp.usdoj.gov/nij/adam/ADAM2003.pdf.

75. Substance Abuse and Mental Health Services Administration, 2003. Drug Abuse Warning Network (DAWN). http://dawninfo.samhsa.gov/old_dawn/pubs_94_02/edpubs/2002final/default.asp#publishedtables.

Chapter 3

1. Office of National Drug Control Policy, 1999. The national drug control strategy: 1999. http://www.ncjrs.org/pdffiles/strat99.pd.52–53.

2. Office of National Drug Control Policy, 2002. The President's national drug control strategy: February 2002. http://www.whitehousedrugpolicy.gov/publications/policy/ndcs02/.11.

3. Harm Reduction Coalition. About HRC. http://www.harmreduction.org/.

4. Committee on Government Reform: Criminal Justice, Drug Policy and Human Resources, 2005. Letter to Honorable Michael O. Leavitt, Secretary, Department of Health and Human Services. http://reform.house.gov/CJDPHR/News/DocumentSingle.aspx?DocumentID=32260 (accessed August 25, 2005).

5. Drug Policy Alliance, 2006. About the Alliance. http://www.drugpolicy.org/about/ (accessed March 20, 2006).

6. Although the term "crack babies" was widely used 5 to 10 years ago, there has never been a syndrome identified in which children exposed to crack or any other

form of cocaine in utero have a specific set of symptoms that can be attributed solely to maternal powder cocaine or crack use.

7. G. R. Hanson, P. J. Venturelli, and A. E. Fleckenstein, 2002. *Drugs and society.* 7th ed. Boston, MA: Jones and Bartlett; Musto, D. F. 1999. *The American disease: Origins of narcotic control.* 3rd ed. New York: Oxford University Press.

8. B. Bullington, L. Bollinger, and T. Shelley, 2004. Trends in European drug policies: A new beginning or more of the same? *Journal of Drug Issues* 34(3): 481–490.

9. Ibid., 484.

10. B. Bullington, 2004. Drug policy reform and its detractors: The United States as the elephant in the closet. *Journal of Drug Issues* 34(3): 696.

11. Ibid.

12. Ibid.

13. Ibid.

14. H. Schmidt-Semisch and P. Bettina, 2002. An alternative to contemporary forms of drugs control. *Journal of Drug Issues* 32(2): 709–720.

15. J. Uitermark, 2004. The origins and future of the Dutch approach towards drugs. *Journal of Drug Issues* 34(3): 511–532.

16. L. Bollinger, 2004. Drug law and policy in Germany and the European community: Recent developments. *Journal of Drug Issues* 34(3): 491–510.

17. N. Dorn, 2004. UK policing of drug traffickers and users: Policy implementation in the contexts of national law, European traditions, international drug conventions, and security after 2001. *Journal of Drug Issues* 34(3): 533–550.

18. Ibid.

19. Ibid.

20. Ibid.

21. J. McGeorge and C. K. Aitken, 1997. Effects of cannabis decriminalization in the Australian Capital Territory on university students' patterns of use. *Journal of Drug Issues* 27(4): 785–793.

22. W. Hall and R. Liccardo Pacula, 2003. *Cannabis use and dependence: Public health and public policy.* Cambridge, UK: Cambridge University Press.

23. Ibid., 163–164.

24. The European School Survey Project on Alcohol and Other Drugs, 2004. The European school survey project on alcohol and other drugs. http://www.espad.org/summary.html (accessed August 30, 2005).

25. Ibid.

26. W. Hall and R. Liccardo Pacula, 2003. *Cannabis use and dependence: Public health and public policy.* Cambridge, UK: Cambridge University Press.

27. B. Bullington, 2004. Drug policy reform and its detractors: The United States as the elephant in the closet. *Journal of Drug Issues* 34(3): 703.

28. Ibid.

29. B. Bullington, L. Bollinger, and T. Shelley, 2004. Trends in European drug policies: A new beginning or more of the same? *Journal of Drug Issues* 34(3): 482.

30. G. R. Hanson, P. J. Venturelli, and A. E. Fleckenstein, 2002. *Drugs and society* (7th ed.). Boston, MA: Jones and Bartlett.

31. National Association of Drug Court Professionals. What is a drug court? http://www.nadcp.org/whatis/ (accessed August 30, 2005).

32. Office National Drug Control Policy, 2005. The President's national drug control strategy: February 2005. http://www.whitehousedrugpolicy.gov/publications/policy/ndcs05/.

33. Center for AIDS Prevention Studies, AIDS Prevention Institute, University of California, San Francisco, 1998. Does HIV needle exchange work? http://www.caps.ucsf.edu/NEPrev.html (accessed August 30, 2005).

34. Ibid.

35. B. Bullington. 2004. Drug policy reform and its detractors: The United States as the elephant in the closet. *Journal of Drug Issues* 34(3): 696.

36. European Monitoring Centre for Drugs and Drug Addiction, 2004. European report on drug consumption rooms. http://www.emcdda.eu.int/index.cfm?fuseaction=public. Content&nNodeID=1327&sLanguageISO=EN.

37. Ibid.

38. Ibid.

39. Ibid.

40. Ibid.

41. Ibid.

42. A. Schroers, 2002. Drug checking: Monitoring the contents of new synthetic drugs. *Journal of Drug Issues* 32(3): 635–646.

43. Ibid.

44. Ibid.

45. J. A. Hogan, K. Reed-Gabrielsen, N. Luna, and D. Grothaus, 2003. *Substance abuse prevention: The intersection of science and practice*. Boston, MA: Allyn & Bacon.

46. W. Hall and R. Liccardo Pacula, 2003. *Cannabis use and dependence: Public health and public policy*. Cambridge, UK: Cambridge University Press.

47. Ibid.

48. J. A. Hogan, K. Reed-Gabrielsen, N. Luna, and D. Grothaus, 2003. *Substance abuse prevention: The intersection of science and practice*. Boston, MA: Allyn & Bacon.

Chapter 4

1. Office of Applied Studies, Substance Abuse and Mental Health Administration, 2005. National Survey on Drug Use and Health. http://oas.samhsa.gov/nsduh/2k4nsduh/2k4Results/2k4Results.htm#lot.

2. Ibid.

3. Ibid.

4. Ibid.

5. Ibid.

6. Office of National Drug Control Policy, 2005. White House Office of National Drug Control Policy National Youth Anti-Drug Media Campaign, Marijuana Initiative. http://www.mediacampaign.org/marijuana/marijuana.html.

7. Office of National Drug Control Policy, 2003. The President's national drug control strategy: February 2003. http://www.whitehousedrugpolicy.gov/publications/policy/ndcs03/stop_use.html.

8. Office of National Drug Control Policy, 2005. White House Drug Czar, research and mental health communities warn parents that marijuana use can lead to depression, suicidal thoughts and schizophrenia. http://www.whitehousedrugpolicy.gov/news/press05/050305.html (accessed September 1, 2005).

9. Ibid.

10. Office of National Drug Control Policy, 2004. Myths & facts: The truth behind 10 popular misperceptions. http://www.whitehousedrugpolicy.gov/publications/marijuana_myths_facts/index.html. 3.

11. Ibid.

12. Office of National Drug Control Policy, 2003. White House Drug Czar, Chair of Congressional Black Caucus Rep. Elijah Cummings and Maryland community leaders discuss harms of "medical marijuana" and warn of danger of marijuana legalization. http://www.whitehousedrugpolicy.gov/news/press03/032403.html (accessed September 1, 2005).

13. Office of National Drug Control Policy, 2005. Statement by the White House Drug Czar about the U.S. Supreme Court's decision regarding so-called medical marijuana. http://www.whitehousedrugpolicy.gov/news/press05/060505.html (accessed September 1, 2005).

14. I could not find this quote in the IOM report. The ONDCP reference is for the IOM report but no page number is given in the reference. I don't doubt that it is there. I just could not find it to document the context of the quote.

15. The Editors, 1995. Deglamorising cannabis. *The Lancet* 346: 1241.

16. L. Zimmer and J. Morgan, 1997. *Marijuana myths, marijuana facts.* New York: The Lindesmith Center.

17. J. E. Joy, S. J. Watson, Jr., and J. A. Benson, Jr. (eds.), 1999. *Marijuana and medicine: Assessing the science base.* Washington, D.C.: National Academy Press.

18. W. Hall and R. Liccardo Pacula, 2003. *Cannabis use and dependence: Public health and public policy.* Cambridge, UK: Cambridge University Press.

19. P. Peretti-Watel, 2005. Cannabis use and dependence: Public health and public policy. *Journal of Epidemiology and Community Health* 2995(59): 435.

20. J. E. Joy, S. J. Watson, Jr., and J. A. Benson, Jr. (eds.), 1999. *Marijuana and medicine: Assessing the science base.* Washington, D.C.: National Academy Press. 7–8.

21. Office of National Drug Control Policy, 2004. *Myths & facts: The truth behind 10 popular misperceptions.* http://www.whitehousedrugpolicy.gov/publications/marijuana_myths_facts/myth1.pdf.11.

22. Marijuana Policy Project, 2006. Another medical marijuana state. http://www.mpp.org/RI_number_11.html (accessed March 20, 2006).

23. Office of National Drug Control Policy, 2005. *The link between marijuana and mental illness: A survey of recent research.* http://www.mediacampaign. org/pdf/marij_mhealth.pdf.

24. University of Maryland, College Park, 2005. Increase in national marijuana admissions driven by increase in criminal justice referrals. *Cesar Fax* 14(32).

25. Ibid.

26. Office of Applied Studies, Substance Abuse and Mental Health Services Administration, 2004. Drug abuse warning network, 2003: Interim national estimates of drug-related emergency department visits. http://dawninfo.samhsa.gov/files/ DAWN_ED_Interim2003.pdf (accessed September 8, 2005).

27. Ibid.

28. The Editors, 2004. Marijuana research: Current restrictions on marijuana research are absurd. *ScientificAmerican.com.* http://www.sciam.com/print_version. cfm?articleID=000A844E-8FBE-119B-8EA483414B7FFE9F (accessed September 8, 2005).

Chapter 5

1. W. J. Hamilton, 2003. Brewing controversy: The story behind the study on underage drinking. MADD Online. http://www.madd.org/news/0,1056,7559_print,00.html.

2. Ibid.

3. This is an annual survey of Americans age 12 and older sponsored by the Substance Abuse and Mental Health Services Administration. The details of the survey were described in Chapter 2.

4. This is an annual survey of 8th, 10th, and 12th graders sponsored by the National Institute on Drug Abuse. The details of the survey were described in Chapter 2.

5. L. D. Johnston, P. M. O'Malley, J. G. Bachman, and J. E. Schulenberg, 2006. Monitoring the future: Table 4, Trends in 30-day prevalence of daily use of various drugs for eighth, tenth, and twelfth graders. http://www.monitoringthefuture. org/data/05data/pr05t4.pdf.

6. National Academy of Sciences, 2004. *Reducing underage drinking: A collective responsibility.* Washington, D.C.: National Academies Press.

7. G. A. Hacker and K. Miller, 2002. NAS Testimony on Underage Drinking. Alcohol Policies Project, Center for Science in the Public Interest. http://www.cspinent. org/booze/NASTestimonyPrint.htm.

8. National Academy of Sciences, 2004. *Reducing underage drinking: A collective responsibility.* Washington, D.C.: National Academies Press.

9. Ibid.

10. Ibid.

11. Ibid.

12. Ibid.

13. Ibid.

14. Office of Applied Studies, Substance Abuse and Mental Health Services Administration, 2003. National Household Survey on Drug Use and Health. Chapter 2: Illicit drug use. http://oas.samhsa.gov/nhsda/2k2nsduh/Results/2k2Results.htm#chap2.

15. The National Center on Addiction and Substance Abuse at Columbia University, 1994. *Cigarettes, alcohol, marijuana: Gateways to illicit drug use.* New York: National Center on Addiction and Substance Abuse at Columbia University.

16. National Academy of Sciences, 2004. *Reducing underage drinking: A collective responsibility.* Washington, D.C.: National Academies Press.

17. Ibid.

18. Office of National Drug Control Policy, 2005. The President's national drug control strategy: FY 2006 budget summary. http://www.whitehousedrugpolicy.gov/publications/policy/06budget/.

19. Office of National Drug Control Policy, 2005. The President's national drug control strategy: FY 2006 budget summary. http://www.whitehousdrugpolicy.gov/publications/policy/06budget/dhhs.pdf.

20. National Institute on Alcohol Abuse and Alcoholism, 2005. Statement by Ting-Kai Li, M.D., Director, National Institute on Alcohol Abuse and Alcoholism, Fiscal Year 2006 President's budget request for the National Institute on Alcohol Abuse and Alcoholism. http://www.niaaa.nih.gov/AboutNIAAA/AdvisoryCouncil/DirectorsReports/Statement3_05.htm.

21. The National Center on Addiction and Substance Abuse at Columbia University, 2003. *The economic value of underage drinking and adult excessive drinking to the alcohol industry.* New York: National Center on Addiction and Substance Abuse at Columbia University.

22. Ibid., 6.

23. Office of Applied Studies, Substance Abuse and Mental Health Services Administration, 2005. *National household survey on drug use and health.* Table H20. http://oas.samhsa.gov/nsduh/2k4nsduh/2k4Results/appH.htm#tabh.20.

24. The National Center on Addiction and Substance Abuse at Columbia University, 2003. *The economic value of underage drinking and adult excessive drinking to the alcohol industry.* New York: National Center on Addiction and Substance Abuse at Columbia University.

25. Ibid.

26. Ibid.

27. Alcohol Policies Project, Center for Science in the Public Interest, 2001. National poll shows "alcopop" drinks lure teens: Groups demand government investigate "starter suds." http://www.cspinet.org/booze/alcopops_press.htm.

28. Alcohol Policies Project, Center for Science in the Public Interest, 2003. Alcoholic-beverage advertising expenditures. Fact sheet. http://www.cspinet.org/booze/FactSheets/AlcAdExp.pdf.

29. The Center on Alcohol Marketing and Youth, 2005. Alcohol advertising and youth. http://camy.org/factsheets/index.php?FactsheetID=1.

30. The Center on Alcohol Marketing and Youth, 2005. Alcohol product commercials overwhelm "responsibility" messages from 2001 to 2003. http://camy.org/press/release.php?ReleaseID=29.

31. W. J. Hamilton, 2003. Brewing controversy: The story behind the study on underage drinking. MADD Online. http://www.madd.org/news/0,1056,7559_print,00.html.

32. Ibid.

33. Center for Responsive Politics, 2005. Political action committees. http://www.opensecrets.org/pacs/index.asp?party=R&cycle=2006 (accessed October 7, 2005).

34. P. Kuntz, 1995. Alcoholic beverage industry lobbies for bill to gut substance abuse agency seen as threat. *Wall Street Journal*. Monday, August 14.

35. Ibid.

36. National Academy of Sciences, 2003. *Reducing underage drinking: A collective responsibility*. Washington, D.C.: National Academies Press.

37. J. Gogek, 2003. The booze lobby: No friend of America's youth. *Washington Post Weekly Edition*. July 21.

38. National Academy of Sciences, 2003. *Reducing underage drinking: A collective responsibility*. Washington, D.C.: National Academies Press.

Chapter 6

1. Office of National Drug Control Policy, 2002. The President's national drug control strategy: February 2002. http://www.whitehousedrugpolicy.gov/publications/policy/ndcs02/.9.

2. J. A. Hogan, K. Reed-Gabrielsen, N. Luna, and D. Grothaus, 2003. *Substance abuse prevention: The intersection of science and practice*. Boston, MA: Allyn & Bacon.

3. Ibid.

4. Ibid.

5. J. D. Hawkins, R. F. Catalano, and J. Y. Miller, 1992. Risk and protective factors for alcohol and other drug problems in adolescence and early adulthood: Implications for substance abuse prevention. *Psychological Bulletin* 112: 64–105.

6. Substance Abuse and Mental Health Services Administration, 2004. SAMHSA unveils strategic prevention framework, $45 million available in state grants. http://alt.samhsa.gov/news/newsreleases/040429nr_spf.htm.

7. J. A. Hogan, K. Reed-Gabrielsen, N. Luna, and D. Grothaus, 2003. *Substance abuse prevention: The intersection of science and practice*. Boston, MA: Allyn & Bacon.

8. Western Region Center for the Application of Prevention Technologies, No date. Developing healthy communities: A risk and protective factor approach to preventing alcohol and other drug abuse. http://captus.samhsa.gov/western/resources/prevmat/DHC-eng.pdf.

9. P. Brounstein, J. Zweig, and S. Gardner, 1998. *Science-based practices in substance abuse: A guide.* Rockville, MD: Center for Substance Abuse Prevention; Substance Abuse and Mental Health Services Administration. 2005. SAMHSA's national registry of evidence-based programs and practices (NREPP). http://modelprograms.samhsa.gov/template.cfm?page=nreppover (accessed September 19, 2005).

10. At the time this manuscript was prepared (November 2005), the 2006 budget had not been approved by Congress and final 2005 budget figures were not available. Before printing the book, the final budget figures for 2005 were included and any changes Congress made in the President's 2006 budget request were noted. The budget figures can be accessed in the ONDCP 2006 NDCS: http://www.whitehousedrugpolicy.gov/publications/policy/07budget/.

11. Office of National Drug Control Policy, 2005. The President's national drug control strategy, FY 2006 budget summary, February 2005.http://www.whitehousedrugpolicy.gov/publications/policy/06budget/dhhs.pdf.

12. Ibid., 25.

13. Office of National Drug Control Policy, 2005. The President's national drug control strategy, FY 2006 budget summary, February 2005. http://www.whitehousedrugpolicy.gov/publications/policy/06budget/justic e.pdf.

14. Office of National Drug Control Policy, 2005. The President's national drug control strategy, FY 2006 budget summary, February 2005. http://www.whitehousedrugpolicy.gov/publications/policy/06budget/education.pdf.

15. Ibid., 18.

16. Ibid., 20.

17. Ibid., 18.

18. R. Yamaguchi, L. D. Johnston, P. M. O'Malley, 2003. The relationship between student illicit drug use and school drug-testing policies. *Journal of School Health* 73: 159.

19. Office of National Drug Control Policy, 2005. The President's national drug control strategy, FY 2006 budget summary, February 2005. http://www.whitehousedrugpolicy.gov/publications/policy/06budget/dhhs.pdf.

20. In the interests of full disclosure: The center I directed has several grants and contracts from this agency, including a contract of approximately $3 million a year from the Center for Substance Abuse Prevention.

21. Office of National Drug Control Policy, 2005. The President's national drug control strategy, FY 2006 budget summary, February 2005. http://www.whitehousedrugpolicy.gov/publications/policy/06budget/dhhs.pdf. CSAP-15.

22. Ibid., 33.

23. Ibid., 33.

24. Ibid., CSAP-1.

25. Ibid., CSAP-6.

26. Ibid., CSAP-6.

27. Ibid., CSAP-7.

28. Another disclosure: The center I directed is the recipient of the Western Center for the Application of Prevention Technologies contract and has had this program since 1997.

29. Office of National Drug Control Policy, 2005. The President's national drug control strategy, FY 2006 budget summary, February 2005. http://www. whitehousedrugpolicy.gov/publications/policy/06budget/dhhs.pdf.CSAP-7.

30. Ibid., 34.

31. Office of National Drug Control Policy, 2005. The President's national drug control strategy, FY 2006 budget summary, February 2005. http://www. whitehousedrugpolicy.gov/publications/policy/06budget/ondc p.pdf.

32. Ibid., 93.

33. Ibid., 96.

34. Office of Management and Budget, 2005. Performance assessment rating tool. http://www.whitehouse.gov/omb/budget/fy2006/pma/agencies.pdf.

35. Office of National Drug Control Policy, 2005. The President's national drug control strategy, FY 2006 budget summary, February 2005. http://www. whitehousedrugpolicy.gov/publications/policy/06budget/ondc p.pdf 93.

36. Ibid., 96.

37. Substance Abuse and Mental Health Services Administration, 2005. SAMHSA model programs: SAMHSA national registry of evidence-based programs and practices (NREPP). http://modelprograms.samhsa.gov/template.cfm?page=nreppover.

38. Alcohol Policies Project, 2003. Fact sheet: Alcoholic-beverage advertising expenditures. http://www.cspinet.org/booze/FactSheets/AlcAdExp.pdf.

39. The 2005 Monitoring the Future results are available for 8th, 10th, and 12th graders but not for college students and young adults. Therefore, the 2004 results were reported in this table for comparison purposes across all groups. It should be noted that there were decreases in annual and lifetime alcohol use from 2004 to 2005 for 8th, 10th, and 12th graders.

40. L. D. Johnston, P. M. O'Malley, J. G. Bachman, and J. E. Schulenberg, 2005. *Monitoring the future national results on adolescent drug use: Overview of key findings, 2004.* NIH Publication No. 05–5726. Bethesda, MD: National Institute on Drug Abuse.

41. Greater Dallas Council on Alcohol & Drug Abuse, 2005. Youth trade drugs at "pharming" parties. http://www.gdcada.org/stories/pharming.htm (accessed March 20, 2006).

42. Office of National Drug Control Policy, 2005. Press release: Youth drug use continues to decline. http://www.whitehousedrugpolicy.gov/NEWS/press05/090805.html.

43. University of Michigan, 2005. Press release: Teen drug use down but progress halts among youngest teens. http://www.monitoringthefuture.org/pressreleases/05drugpr.pdf.

44. S. Suo, 2004. Lobbyists and loopholes. *The Oregonian.* http://www.oregonlive.com/special/oregonian/meth/stories/index.ssf?/oregonian/meth/1004_lobbyistsandloopholes.html.

45. S. M. Friedman, 2005. Inflation calculator. http://www.westegg.com/inflation/.

46. V. Colman and B. Suiter, 2002. Tobacco prevention and control in Washington State: A comprehensive report. *Northwest Public Health.* Fall/Winter: 6–9.

47. Center for Substance Abuse Prevention, No date. Synar amendment: Protecting the nation's youth from nicotine addiction. http://prevention.samhsa.gov/tobacco/.

48. J. J. Wilson, 1999. Summary of the Attorneys General Master Tobacco Settlement Agreement, National Conference of State Legislators. http://academic.udayton.edu/health/syllabi/tobacco/summary.htm.

49. American Legacy Foundation, 2004. Building a world where young people reject tobacco and anyone can stop smoking. http://www.americanlegacy.org/americanlegacy/skins/alf/display.aspx?Action=display_page&mode=User&ModuleID=8cde2e88–3052–448c-893d-d0b4b14b31c4&ObjectID=e203e4bd-d5ac-4d5b-90ce-cfbfaf0e3db8.

50. M. C. Farrelly, K. C. Davis, M. L. Haviland, P. Messeri, and C. G. Healton, 2005. Evidence of a dose-response relationship between "truth" antismoking ads and youth smoking prevalence. *American Journal of Public Health* 95(3): 425–431.

51. There is a great deal of controversy regarding the continuing efforts of the tobacco industry to market their product to underage smokers through outlets such as magazines and product placement in movies. This continued marketing may be contributing to the diminishing decreases in youth smoking in the past couple of years. In fact, there were increases in the rates for 12th graders, college students, and young adults from 2003 to 2004 (see Table 2.6).

52. American Legacy Foundation, 2004. Building a world where young people reject tobacco and anyone can stop smoking. http://www.americanlegacy.org/americanlegacy/skins/alf/display.aspx?Action=display_page&mode=User&ModuleID=8cde2e88–3052–448c-893d-d0b4b14b31c4&ObjectID=e203e4bd-d5ac-4d5b-90ce-cfbfaf0e3db8.

53. Centers for Disease Control, 1998. Guidelines for school health programs to prevent tobacco use and addiction. http://wonder.cdc.gov/wonder/prevguid/m0026213/m0026213.asp.

54. D. M. Gorman, 1998. The irrelevance of evidence in the development of school-based drug prevention policy, 1986–1996. *Evaluation Review* 22(1): 118–146.

55. G. J.Botvin, E. Dusenbury, S. Baker, E. James-Ortiz, E. Botvin, and J. Kemer, 1992. Smoking prevention among urban minority youth: Assessing effects on outcome and mediating variables. *Health Psychology* 11: 290–299.

56. American Legacy Foundation, 2004. Building a world where young people reject tobacco and anyone can stop smoking. http://www.americanlegacy.org/americanlegacy/skins/alf/display.aspx?Action=display_page&mode=User&ModuleID=8cde2e88-3052-448c-893d-d0b4b14b31c4&ObjectID=e203e4bd-d5ac-4d5b-90ce-cfbfaf0e3db8.

57. P. Brounstein, J. Zweig, and S. Gardner, 1998. *Science-based practices in substance abuse: A guide*. Rockville, MD: Center for Substance Abuse Prevention.

58. Ibid.

59. M. Klitzner, 1998. *Integrating environmental change theory into prevention practice*. Vienna, VA: Klitzner and Associates.

Chapter 7

1. The term "client" or "patient" may be used depending on one's orientation. I prefer "client."

2. Substance use disorders are defined by criteria in the *Diagnostic and statistical manual of mental disorders* developed by the American Psychiatric Association. There are substance abuse and substance dependence disorders, with the former being more severe than the later.

3. At the time this manuscript was prepared (November 2005), the 2006 budget had not been approved by Congress and the final 2005 budget figures were not available. Before printing the book, the final budget figures for 2005 were included and any changes Congress made in the President's 2006 budget request were noted. The budget figures can be accessed in the ONDCP 2006 NDCS: http://www.whitehousedrugpolicy.gov/publications/policy/07budget/.

4. Office of National Drug Control Policy, 2005. The President's national drug control strategy, FY 2006 budget summary, February 2005. http://www.whitehousedrugpolicy.gov/publications/policy/06budg et/dhhs.pdf.

5. Office of National Drug Control Policy, 2005. The President's national drug control strategy, FY 2006 budget summary, February 2005. http://www.whitehousedrugpolicy.gov/publications/policy/06budg et/justice.pdf.

6. Ibid.

7. Ibid., 80.

8. Ibid., 81.

9. Office of National Drug Control Policy, 2005. The President's national drug control strategy, FY 2006 budget summary, February 2005. http://www.whitehousedrugpolicy.gov/publications/policy/06budg et/veterans_affairs.pdf.

10. Office of National Drug Control Policy, 2005. The President's national drug control strategy, FY 2006 budget summary, February 2005. http://www.whitehousedrugpolicy.gov/publications/policy/06budg et/dhhs.pdf.

11. The center I directed has three programs funded by the Center for Substance Abuse Treatment.

12. One of the programs in the center I directed would have reduced funding if this is approved.

13. This does not represent discrete individuals because if a person is admitted more than once in a calendar year, he/she would be counted every time he/she was admitted.

14. Office of Applied Studies, Substance Abuse and Mental Health Services Administration, 2006. Treatment Episode Data Set (TEDS) Highlights—2004: National admissions to substance abuse treatment services. http://wwwdasis.samhsa.gov/teds04/tedshigh2k4.pdf.

15. Ibid.

16. Ibid.

17. Ibid.

18. Ibid.

19. National Institute on Drug Abuse, 1999. *Principles of drug addiction treatment: A research-based guide*, p. 3. Washington, D.C.: National Institute of Health.

20. D. Gerstein, R. Datta, J. Ingels, R. Fredson, K. Rasinski, S. Schildhaus, K. Talley, et al., 1997. *National treatment improvement evaluation study: Final report.* Washington, D.C.: U.S. Department of Health and Human Services.

21. Z. Zhang, P. D. Friedmann, and D. R. Gerstein, 2003. Does retention matter: Treatment duration and improvement in drug use. *Addiction* 98(5): 673–684.

22. National Institute on Drug Abuse, 2005. NIDA notes: Economists offer program for costing out drug abuse treatment. http://www.nida.nih.gov/NIDA_notes/NNvol19N5/Economists.ht ml.

23. National Institute on Drug Abuse, 1997. NIDA notes: Study sheds new light on the state of drug abuse treatment nationwide. http://www.drugabuse.gov/NIDA_Notes/NNVol12N5/Study.html.

24. M. L. Predergast, D. Podus, E. C., and D. Urada, 2003. The effectiveness of drug abuse treatment: A meta-analysis of comparison group studies. *Drug and Alcohol Dependence* 67(1): 53–72.

25. S. Belenko, N. Patapis, and M. T. French, 2005. *Economic benefits of drug treatment: A critical review of the evidence for policy makers.* University of Pennsylvania: Treatment Research Institute.

26. Office of Applied Studies, Substance Abuse and Mental Health Services Administration, 2004. National Household Survey on Drug Use and Health, Chapter 7: Substance dependence, abuse, and treatment. http://www.oas.samhsa.gov/nhsda/2k3nsduh/2k3Results.htm#7.2.

27. Ibid.

28. Ibid.

29. A. T. McLellan, D. C. Lewis, C. P. O'Brien, and H. D. Kleber, 2000. Drug dependence, a chronic mental illness: Implications for treatment, insurance, and outcome evaluation. *JAMA* 284: 1689–1695.

30. Faces and Voices of Recovery, No date. Home page. http://www.facesandvoicesofrecovery.org/main/index.php.

31. E. M. Jellinek, 1960. *The disease concept of alcoholism.* New Haven, CT: Hillhouse Press.

32. G. L. Fisher, and T. C. Harrison, 2005. *Substance abuse: Information for school counselors, social workers, therapists, and counselors.* 3rd ed. Boston, MA: Pearson Education.

33. Alcoholics Anonymous does not take any official position on the disease concept or any other controversial issue. The disease concept is associated with Alcoholics Anonymous because many participants in this program subscribe to the disease concept.

34. G. L. Fisher and T. C. Harrison, 2005. *Substance abuse: Information for school counselors, social workers, therapists, and counselors.* 3rd ed. Boston, MA: Pearson Education.

35. H. Fingarette, 1988. *Heavy drinking: The myth of alcoholism as a disease.* Berkeley, CA: University of California.

36. A. T. McLellan, D. C. Lewis, C. P. O'Brien, and H. D. Kleber, 2000. Drug dependence, a chronic medical illness: Implications for treatment, insurance, and outcomes evaluation. *JAMA* 284: 1689–1695.

37. Ibid., 1694.

38. Ibid.

39. Center for Substance Abuse Treatment, 2005. *Substance abuse treatment for persons with co-occurring disorders.* Treatment Improvement Protocol (TIP) Series 42. DHHS Publication No. (SMA) 05-3992. Rockville, MD: Substance Abuse and Mental Health Services Administration.

40. Ibid.

41. D. J. Rohsenow, R. Corbett, and D. Devine, 1988. Molested as children: A hidden contribution to substance abuse? *Journal of Substance Abuse* 39: 13–18.

42. Center for Substance Abuse Treatment, 2005. *Substance abuse treatment for persons with co-occurring disorders.* Treatment Improvement Protocol (TIP) Series 42. DHHS Publication No. (SMA) 05–3992. Rockville, MD: Substance Abuse and Mental Health Services Administration.

43. American Psychiatric Association, 2000. *Diagnostic and statistical manual of mental disorders.* 4th ed., text revision. Washington, D.C.: American Psychiatric Association.

44. Ibid., 706.

45. W. M. Compton, K. P. Conway, F. S. Stinson, J. D. Colliver, and B. F. Grant, 2005. Prevalence, correlates, and comorbidity of DSM-IV Antisocial personality syndromes and alcohol and specific drug use disorders in the United States: Results from the National Epidemiologic Survey on Alcohol and Related Conditions. *Journal of Clinical Psychiatry* 66: 677–685.

46. P. W. Long, 1990. Antisocial personality disorder. Internet mental health. http://www.mentalhealth.com/rx/p23-pe04.html.

47. D. W. Black, 2000. Treatment for antisocial personality disorder. Psych Central. http://psychcentral.com/library/asp_tx.htm.

48. J. W. Dilley, 2004. Antisocial personality disorder. *Medlineplus medical encyclopedia.* http://www.nlm.nih.gov/medlineplus/ency/article/000921.htm.

49. A. T. McLellan, D. C. Lewis, C. P. O'Brien, and H. D. Kleber, 2000. Drug dependence, a chronic mental illness: Implications for treatment, insurance, and outcome evaluation. *JAMA* 284: 1689–1695.

50. L. C. Sobell, J. A. Cunningham, and M. B. Sobell, 1996. Recovery from alcohol problems with or without treatment: Prevalence in two population surveys. *American Journal of Public Health* 86: 966–972.

51. Office of Applied Studies, Substance Abuse and Mental Health Services Administration, 2005. Treatment Episode Data Set (TEDS) Highlights—2003: National admissions to substance abuse treatment services. http://wwwdasis.samhsa. gov/teds03/2003_teds_highlights.pdf.

52. U.S. Department of Housing and Urban Development, 1999. Homelessness: Programs and people they serve. Interagency Council on the Homeless. http://www.huduser.org/publications/homeless/homelessness/ch_2c.html#table2.4.

53. G. L. Fisher, and T. C. Harrison, 2005. *Substance abuse: Information for school counselors, social workers, therapists, and other counselors.* 3rd ed. Boston, MA: Pearson Education.

54. K. Humphreys, S. Wing, D. McCarty, J. Chappel, L. Gallant, B. Haberle, A. T. Horvath, et al., 2004. Self-help organizations for alcohol and drug problems: Toward evidence-based practice and policy. *Journal of Substance Abuse Treatment* 26: 154.

55. These labels will help the reader remember the situation for each person.

Chapter 8

1. Office of National Drug Control Policy, 2005. Bush cabinet officials highlight administration anti-meth programs. http://www.whitehousedrugpolicy.gov/news/press05/081805.html.

2. S. Suo, 2005. Drug czar, aide face meth criticism. *The Oregonian.* September 29, 2005.http://www.oregonlive.com/news/oregonian/index.ssf?/base/front_page/1127991476181420.xml&coll=7&thispage=1 (accessed October 13, 2005).

3. Office of National Drug Control Policy, 2006. National drug control strategy: FY 2007 budget summary. http://www.whitehousedrugpolicy.gov/publications/policy/07budget/partii_funding_tables.pdf.

4. At the time this manuscript was prepared (November 2005), the 2006 budget had not been approved by Congress and final 2005 budget figures were not available. Before printing the book, the final budget figures for 2005 were included and any changes Congress made in the President's 2006 budget request were noted. The budget figures can be accessed in the ONDC 2006 NDCS: http://www.whitehousedrugpolicy.gov/publications/policy/07budget/.

5. Office of National Drug Control Policy, 2005. The President's national drug control strategy: FY 2006 budget summary. http://www.whitehousedrugpolicy.gov/publications/policy/06budget/state.pdf.

6. Ibid., 102.

7. Ibid., 100.

8. Office of National Drug Control Policy, 2005. The President's national drug control strategy: FY 2006 budget summary. http://www.whitehousedrugpolicy.gov/publications/policy/06budget/defense.pdf.

9. Ibid., 13.

10. Office of National Drug Control Policy, 2005. The President's national drug control strategy: FY 2006 budget summary. http://www.whitehousedrugpolicy. gov/publications/policy/06budget/homeland_security.pdf.

11. Ibid., 51.

12. Ibid., 46.

13. Ibid., 40.

14. Office of National Drug Control Policy, 2005. The President's national drug control strategy: FY 2006 budget summary. http://www.whitehousedrugpolicy. gov/publications/policy/06budget/justice.pdf.

15. Ibid., 69.

16. Ibid., 62.

17. Office of National Drug Control Policy, 2005. The President's national drug control strategy. Chapter III: Disrupting the market: Attacking the economic basis of the drug trade, pp. 39–41. http://www.whitehousedrugpolicy. gov/publications/policy/ndcs05/index.html.

18. Office of National Drug Control Policy, 1998. The national drug control strategy. Chapter III: Strategic goals and objectives. http://www.ncjrs.org/ondcppubs/ pdf/strat_pt2.pdf.23.

19. Pittsburgh Post-Gazette, 2005. Editorial: Junk this plan/The U.S. drug war in Colombia isn't working. *Pittsburgh Post-Gazette* May 2. http://www.post-gazette.com/ pg/05122/497563.stm. (accessed October 14, 2005).

20. L. Samuels, and L. Iliff, 2005. Analysts say Mexico drug fight a failure. *Dallas Morning News* July 4. http://www.dallasnews.com/s/dws/dn/ latestnews/stories/070405dnintdrugwar.6f872939.html (accessed October 14, 2005).

21. C. A. Youngers, and E. Rosin (eds.), 2004. *Drugs and democracy in Latin America: The impact of U.S. policy* 2.

22. United Nations Office on Drugs and Crime, 2005. *2005 world drug report.* Executive summary. http://www.unodc.org/unodc/en/world_drug_report.html.

23. Ibid., 5.

24. Ibid., 8.

25. Ibid., 5.

26. Ibid.

27. Ibid.

28. Ibid.

29. United Nations Office on Drugs and Crime, 2005. *2005 world drug report.* Chapter 2: Estimating the value of illicit drug markets. http://www.unodc.org/pdf/ WDR_2005/volume_1_web.pdf.

30. Ibid.

31. Office of National Drug Control Policy, 2001. *What America's users spend of illegal drugs: 1988–2000.* http://www.whitehousedrugpolicy.gov/publications/ pdf/american_users_spend_2002.pdf.

32. United Nations Office on Drugs and Crime, 2005. *2005 world drug report*. Executive Summary. http://www.unodc.org/unodc/en/world_drug_report.html.

33. 60 Minutes, 2005. Afghanistan: Addicted to heroin. October 16. http://www.cbsnews.com/stories/2005/10/14/60minutes/main946648.shtml.

34. C. A. Youngers and E. Rosin (eds.), 2004. *Drugs and democracy in Latin America: The impact of U.S. policy.* http://www.wola.org/publications/ddhr_exec_sum_brief.pdf.12–13.

35. Ibid., 13.

Chapter 9

1. Nicotine is clearly an addictive drug with mind-altering properties. It is not being included here to maintain the focus on drugs with serious consequences in many areas, not just physical health. This is not meant to minimize the tremendous damage that smoking causes.

2. National Academy of Sciences, 2004. *Reducing underage drinking: A collective responsibility*. Washington, D.C.: National Academies Press.

3. Ibid., 240–241.

4. The Tax Foundation, 2005. Federal excise tax collections: 1940–2004. http://www.taxfoundation.org/research/show/240.html (accessed October 20, 2005).

5. M. F. Fleming, M. P. Mundt, M. T. French, L. Baier-Manwell, E. A. Stauffacher, and K. F. Lawton-Berry, 2002. Brief physician advice for problem drinkers: Long-term efficacy and benefit-cost analysis. *Alcoholism: Clinical and Experimental Research* 26: 36–43; A. I. Wilk, N. M. Jensen, and T. C. Havighurst, 1997. Meta-analysis of randomized control trials addressing brief interventions in heavy alcohol drinkers. *Journal of General Internal Medicine* 12: 274–283.

6. National Institutes of Health, 1998. NIH guide: Effectiveness of strategies for preventing DUI recidivism. PAS-99–023 http://grants.nih.gov/grants/guide/pa-files/PAS-99–023.html (accessed October 24, 2005).

Index

alcoholism and drug addiction, 125–45; as chronic conditions, 135–39, 141, 143, 144, 171–72, 174; children of alcoholics/addicts, 101, 103; criminality related to, 162–63, 174–75; disease model of, 134–35, 139, 143; genetics as a casual factor in, 135–36; numbers of people with, 35, 88–89, 158; public health concept of 133–34, 162–63, 172, 174; recovery from, 125; risk factors for, 101–105, 115–16; treatment for. *See* treatment

Alcohol Policies Project, 92

American Bar Association, x

American Legacy Foundation, 121–22, 169. *See also* tobacco

American Lung Association, 122. *See also* tobacco

American Medical Association, x, 134

American Psychiatric Association, 134, 137

amphetamine, 55

Amsterdam, 60

Andean Counterdrug Initiative, 16, 148–49

Andean Region, 14–15, 58

Anti-Drug Abuse Acts, 5, 87

anti-social personality disorder, 137–38, 142–44, 162–63, 174–75. *See also* treatment, and co-occurring mental disorders

Arrestee Drug Abuse Monitoring Program (ADAM), 23, 46, 50–51

Aruba, 16

Ativan, 55, 85. *See also* prescription drugs

Australia, 61

Automated Tracking Initiative, 17

barbiturates, 55, 59

Bayer Corporation, 58

Belgium, 61

Bennett, William, 5, 6

Bias, Len, 5

Block Grant, 12–13, 15–16, 108, 112, 120, 128–29, 133

Boggs Act, 58

Bolivia, 16, 154, 157

Border Patrol, 14, 16

Britain, 58, 60, 62

British Medical Journal, 72

Brown, Lee, 5

buprenorphine, 63, 172, 174

Bureau of Prisons, 127

Bureau of the Census, 49

Bush Administration, 1–2, 6–7, 16, 19, 31, 36, 54, 57, 84, 139, 147, 152–53

Bush, President George Herbert Walker, 5

Bush, President George W., 6–7, 25, 27, 37, 129

caffeine, 55

Canada, 44, 60, 164

cannabinoids. *See* marijuana

cannabis. *See* marijuana

Caribbean, 14, 16

Carter, President Jimmy, 4

Catalano, Richard, 102

Center for Science in the Public Interest, 92

Center for Substance Abuse Prevention, xiv, 93, 102, 108–10, 112–14, 120

Center for Substance Abuse Treatment, 3, 63, 128–29, 131, 133, 136–37

Center on Addiction and Substance Abuse, 90–91

Center on Alcohol Marketing and Youth, 92

Centers for Disease Control, 34, 121

Centers for the Application of Prevention Technologies, 109–10, 114

Central America, 5, 13, 165

China, 58

cigarettes. *See* tobacco

drug abuse treatment. *See* treatment
Drug Abuse Warning Network
    (DAWN), 47–48, 50–51, 81
drug addiction. *See* alcoholism and drug
    addiction
drug addicts. *See* alcoholism and drug
    addiction
drug courts, 13–14, 16–18, 63–64, 81,
    127–28, 172
Drug Czars, 2, 4–5, 83. *See also*
    McCaffrey, Barry; Walters, John
drug dependence. *See* alcoholism and
    drug addiction
Drug Enforcement Administration
    (DEA), 4, 6, 11, 13–18, 22, 42,
    150–51, 166
drug eradication. *See* supply reduction,
    eradication
Drug-Free Communities Act and
    Drug-Free Communities Support
    Program, 14–18, 110–11,
    114
Drug Intervention Program, 15–16
Drug Policy Alliance, 56–57, 71
Drug Policy Foundation, 56
drug-related arrests. *See* alcohol and drug
    abuse, relationship to arrests and
    crime
Drug Seizure System, 41
drug testing, 13, 15, 18, 56, 101, 107–8,
    112–13
drug trafficking. *See* supply reduction,
    drug trafficking
DUI, 123, 142, 168, 170
Dutch. *See* Netherlands

Eastern Pacific, 16
ecstasy, 66, 147, 158; age of first use,
    33–34
Ecuador, 16
Egyptians, 58
Elders, Jocelyn, 3
Europe, 43, 171

European Monitoring Centre for Drugs
    and Drug Addiction, 65
evidenced-based practices. *See*
    prevention, evidence-based practices
    in; treatment,
evidence-based practices in
excise taxes. *See* alcohol, excise taxes;
    tobacco, excise taxes
Executive Order No. 12880, 5

faith-based organizations and programs,
    17, 119, 128, 142–45
Federal-wide Drug Seizure System
    (FDSS), 41–43
Financial and Money Laundering,
    Initiative, 17
FIREBIRD, 15–16
Food and Drug Administration, 168
Ford, President Gerald, 4
Forward Operating Locations, 15–16
Fox, President Vicente, 153
France, 62

Gamblers Anonymous, 140
generalized anxiety disorder. *See*
    treatment, and co-occurring mental
    disorders
Germany, 65–66
Gonzales, Attorney General Alberto, 147
Government Performance and Results
    Act (GPRA), 105–106, 127
Greeks, 58

hallucinogens, 55, 59, 67; age of first
    use, 33–34
harm reduction, xi, 3, 53–57, 62–67,
    163, 169–73; argument against,
    53–54; drug checking, 66; drug
    consumption rooms, 65–66, 171–73,
    175–76; drug courts. *See* drug courts;
    heroin distribution programs, 64–65;
    needle exchange programs, 47, 56–57,
    64, 171; opiate substitution therapies,

marijuana (*cont.*)

for dependence on, 129; age of first use, 27, 32–35; arguments on dangers of, 72–73; arguments against dangers of, 73–74; as a gateway drug, 76, 82; availability of, 22, 39, 43–45, 66, 154, 157; barriers to research of, 83; categorization as Schedule I drug, 55, 83, 173; compared to alcohol, 80–81, 88; decriminalization of, 4, 6, 55, 57, 60–62, 173; emergency room visits related to, 47–48, 81–82; eradication of, 5, 13, 22, 150, 166; legalization of, xiii–xiv, 67–68, 173; medical uses of, xiii, 2, 4, 6, 54, 56, 73, 76–78, 85–86, 173; objective information regarding, 75–82; ONDCP activities to prevent use of, 17, 71–72, 110; physical effects of chronic use, 78–79; price and purity of, 22, 39–40, 45; psychological effects of, 72–73, 76, 79–80; relationship to other drug use and addiction, 31–32, 90, 103; strategies to reduce harm caused by, 14, 173; supply reduction efforts, 13, 153; THC content of, 39–40; treatment admissions, 81; use of by adults, 31, 36, 71; use of by college students and young adults, 27, 29, 32–33, 71, 85, 117–18; use of by youth, 14, 27 29, 32–33, 37, 62, 71, 85, 89, 113, 117–18; withdrawal from, 76, 80–81

Marijuana Initiative, 71–72

Marijuana Policy Project, 71

Marijuana Tax Act, 58

Master Tobacco Settlement Agreement, 120–21

McCaffrey, Barry, 2, 5–6, 16, 60, 87, 152, 162

Media Campaign, 3, 14–17, 92–93, 110–16, 121, 124, 169

mescaline, 55. *See also* hallucinogens

methadone, 57, 63–64, 126, 142–45, 172–73. *See also* harm reduction, opiate substitution therapies; treatment

methamphetamine, 15, 55, 67, 150, 165–66, 171; availability of, 15, 22, 41–42, 44–45, 147, 158; emergency room visits related to, 48, 82; price and purity of, 22, 39–40, 45; production of, 22, 38, 40, 41–42, 44, 119, 157, 166

methylphenidate. *See* Ritalin

Mexico, 5, 11, 15, 42–44, 147, 152–54, 164

minor tranquilizers. *See* prescription drugs

Mobile Enforcement Teams, 13

money laundering. *See* supply reduction, money laundering

Monitoring the Future Survey (MTF), 21, 24–30, 32–33, 37–38, 89, 107, 111, 117

morphine, 58, 64

narcoterrorism, 165

narcotic pain relief drugs. *See* prescription drugs

Narcotics Anonymous (NA), 126, 134, 140–42

Narcotics Control Act of 1956, 58–59

National Academy of Sciences, 75, 88; report on underage drinking, 90, 93–97, 164, 168

National Beer Wholesalers Association, 93–94

National Drug Control Strategy (NDCS), x, xiii, xiv, xv, 2–3, 5, 10, 72, 84, 88, 99, 116, 119, 120, 126, 162, 164; barriers to progress on, 4; budgets for, 7–9, 148; components of, 11–18, 119–20; components of new, 167–75; demand reduction in, 7, 12–18, 100–1, 105–12, 127–29, 132,

139, 157–58,161. *See also* prevention; treatment; evidence of failure of initiatives, 18–51, 155, 161; guiding principles for new, 162–63, 165; harm reduction, decriminalization, legalization, view of in, 53–55, 57, 60, 63–64, 161; initiatives in annual strategies, 12–18; supply reduction in, 12–18, 66, 148–52, 156–57, 161. *See also* supply reduction; supply reduction vs. demand reduction, 6, 7; targets in, 18–51, 87

pain relief drugs. *See* prescription drugs
Panama, 5
Parents Drug Corps Program, 16
Percodan, 55. *See also* prescription drugs
Peru, 14, 16, 154
peyote, 55. *See also* hallucinogens
pharming, 118
Pittsburgh Post-Gazette, 153
Plan Colombia. *See* Colombia, Plan
    Colombia
Platzspitz park, 62
poppy. *See* supply reduction, eradication
post-traumatic stress disorder. *See*
    treatment, and co-occurring mental
    disorders
prescription drugs, 75, 85–86, 118, 158;
    age of first use, 34; use of by youth,
    118. *See also* illicit drugs, specific
    prescription drugs (e.g., Darvocet,
    Valium)
prevention: activities in the NDCS,
    105–12; definition of, 7; efforts to
    limit tobacco use, 119–23;
    environmental strategies in, 122–23,
    168–70; evidence-based practices in,
    105, 109, 113–14; evidence on
    effectiveness of federal initiatives,
    105–12, 114; impact of alcohol
    marketing, 116; impact of
    experimentation by youth, 117–18;
    impact of pharmaceutical marketing,
    118–19; national outcome measures,
    108–9, 113; Programs of Regional
    and National Significance, 109–10;
    rationale for, 99; reasons why
    effectiveness not demonstrated,
    112–19; strategies, 100–1; target
    populations for, 101; strategies to
    improve, 123–24, 167–69. *See also*
    Decision Support System; Life Skills
    Training; Media Campaign; National
    Registry of Evidence-based Programs
    and Practices; risk and protective

factors; State Incentive Grants;
    Strategic Prevention Framework State
    Incentive Grants
PRIDE Survey, 21, 38
Program Assessment Rating Tool
    (PART), 105–13, 127–29, 148–51
pseudoephedrine, 119, 147, 158. *See also*
    methamphetamine
psilocybin, 55. *See also* hallucinogens

RAND Corporation's Drug Policy
    Research Center, 75
Reagan administration, 162
Reagan, Nancy, 5
Reagan, President Ronald, 5
recovery. *See* alcoholism and drug
    addiction, recovery from
Rehr, David, 94
risk and protective factors, 101–5, 109,
    112, 114–16, 124, 163,
    167–68
Ritalin, 55, 118

Safe and Drug-Free Schools and
    Communities Program, 12–14,
    16–18, 107
School Coordinator Initiative, 16
Scientific American, 83
screening and brief interventions, 18,
    96, 169
Senate Subcommittee on Substance
    Abuse and Mental Health Services,
    Committee on Health, Education,
    Labor and Pensions, 97
Single Convention on Narcotic Drugs,
    59
Single State Authority, 108, 128–29
smoking. *See* tobacco
Souder, Representative Mark, 56–57
South America, 41, 43, 165
Southeast Asia, 43, 165
Southwest Asia, 43, 165
Southwest Border, 12–14

tranquilizers. *See* prescription drugs
Treasury Department, 14
treatment: abstinence models of, 139, 144, 172; access and retention in, 132–33; activities in the NDCS, 7, 127–29; admissions to public sector programs, 129–30; and co-occurring mental disorders, 133, 136–38, 143–44, 174; and special populations, 126, 128; and criminal justice systems, 129, 130, 139; description of, 126–27; effectiveness of, 131–32; evidence-based practices in, 128; in new NDCS, 173–75; length of stay in, 130–33, 173; Minnesota model of, 134; multiple admissions to, 129, 139, 172; need for, 132, 169; Programs of Regional and National Significance, 128–29; public sector, 126–27, 173–75; relapse following, 133, 135, 138–39, 144, 175; Residential Substance Abuse Treatment, 16, 127–28; settings for, 126, 130–32, 173–74; spirituality as a component of, 140–41; stigma as barrier to, 132–34 strategies to improve, 144–45, 173–75
tuberculosis, 23, 46–47, 64

U.S./Mexican border, 6,
underage drinking, 87–92, 107, 112, 162; alcohol industry role in, 92–93, 161, 168; and alcohol advertising, 92–93, 168; and illicit drug use, 89, 90–91, 103, 168; and youth-oriented alcohol products, 92; binge drinking by young people, 89–90; federal expenditures to prevent, 6, 91; harm

caused by, 90–91; recommendations from the National Academy of Sciences regarding, 94–97, 168; social and economic costs of, 90; value to alcohol industry, 91–92. *See also* alcohol
Underage Drinking Prevention Program, 106
United Kingdom. *See* Britain
United Nations Office on Drugs and Crime, 154
University of Queensland, 75

Valium, 55, 85. *See also* prescription drugs
Veterans Health Administration, 12–13, 128
violence prevention. *See* prevention
Violent Crime Control and Law Enforcement Act of 1994, 5

Wall Street Journal, 93
Walters, John, 2, 6, 60, 72–73, 75, 77, 84, 147, 152–53
War on Drugs, 2, 4, 147, 162
Washington Office on Latin America, 154, 156
Washington Post, 16
Weed and Seed, 106
World Drug Report, 154–55

Xanax, 55, 85. *See also* prescription drugs

Youth Risk Behavior Surveillance Survey (YRBSS), 20, 23, 34, 48–49
Youth Substance Abuse Prevention Initiative (YSAPI), 14–15, 17, 71, 110
Youth Treatment Initiative, 14

About the Author

GARY L. FISHER is Founder, Director and Professor at the Center for the Application of Substance Abuse Technologies at the University of Nevada at Reno. Earlier a Professor of Counseling and Educational Psychology, he is the author of a textbook on substance abuse counseling that is now in its third edition. Fisher's career has spanned 31 years and includes work as a private practice clinician and in public schools as a psychologist. The center he directs now in Reno provides drug and alcohol counselors and prevention specialists with state-of-the-art training.